Dear Sanjay:

Hopefully, this

to saving lives from heart attacks.

Best regards,

Sameer.

Preparing for Your Heart Attack…And Surviving It

SAMEER MEHTA MD

This book is lovingly dedicated to my son, Kabir, whose persistent encouragement has made this endeavor possible.

CONTENTS

FOREWORD

It is a pleasure to introduce Dr. Sameer Mehta's book, "Preparing for Your Heart Attack" – the message is incomplete without the subtitle, "And Surviving It". Ignore this book at your own peril. Or, instead, be wise and spend a delightful 4 hours reading this little masterpiece and get a real shot at surviving a heart attack. Not a bad investment of 4 hours of your time and $14.99!

I have known Sameer since he was a colleague at Miami Heart Institute in 1989. He was a passionate Interventional Cardiologist then, but was honing his multiple talents of an academician, researcher and educator. We lost individual contact for a while though I remained conversant of Sameer's work in saving lives from heart attacks. His contributions to Medicine are profound and he has single handedly created the specialty of a STEMI Cardiologist. It is virtually impossible for another cardiologist to catch up with his volume of individual STEMI procedures – whereas most interventional cardiologists perform an average of 11 STEMI procedures each year, Sameer has been averaging >200. Mind you, each of these procedure demands an immediate cessation of your activity. Translated, you have no life.

Foremost, his individual sacrifices as well as those of his family judge Sameer's contributions. It is truly amazing to fathom the breadth of his global endeavors in heart attack care. Creating heart attack programs in thirty countries and conducting an international seminar for twenty years on heart attacks is stupendous work. I also remain fascinated by the creating of the LATIN Telemedicine program that now provides an umbrella of heart attack coverage to more than 100 million patients.

You will not be disappointed reading this book. Instead, you will learn much about what causes a heart attack and how you can prevent it. Modern advances in angioplasty can save most lives from heart attacks but that mandates the initial recognition of symptoms by you. This fundamental and critical principal is the essence of this book. You will unambiguously understand whether you are vulnerable to having a heart attack. You also have a practical checklist of decision points – all these will save your life. Not only your life, it will save the lives of your loved ones too. My favorite chapter of the book is the one addressing heart attacks in the elderly. I constantly worry about my elder relatives and I picked up pearls about how to deal with the situation of their ever having a heart attack.

In the section of prevention, there is a large section about life style modification, including diet. This chimes in with my life's work on this topic and my very popular, South Beach Diet.

Go ahead; make your day – read this book. Get ahead of the game – give yourself a real shot of surviving a heart attack

Arthur Agatson, MD

Miami Beach, Florid

PREFACE

Wherever the art of medicine is loved, there is also a love of humanity.

Hippocrates

This crazy title was adapted after vacillating in my head for years. It arose from simple observations after watching financial planners – plan for your retirement, plan for your children's education, and so forth. We spend an enormous amount of time planning these important issues, getting consultants to advice on this too. But have we planned to manage what may be the most important event in our lives – death from a heart attack? In the last 15 years of my extraordinary career, I sincerely believe that I have completely unlocked the secrets of not only surviving a heart attack, but also preventing it. These two critical messages, of surviving a heart attack and preventing the next one, form the essential decree for this book. Lest this critical subject not catch your urgent attention, let me cite statistics. Most of us, men and women, will die from a heart attack! The real tragedy is that almost all these deaths can be averted by comprehensively understanding the modern treatment of heart attacks and about the rational approaches to prevent it.

My foray into heart attack management originated after several years of practice as an expert interventional cardiologist, whereby I performed angioplasty for treating coronary artery disease.

This book is written for the layperson, and I will begin this task by demystifying   some scientific terms. The remarkable procedure of angioplasty, either using balloons, cutting devices, or metallic scaffolds known as stents, unclogs one of the three coronary arteries and restores blood to the heart muscle. The modern definition of angioplasty using a multitude of these devices are known as PCI or percutaneous coronary intervention. When specifically used to treat heart attacks, PCI is known as Primary PCI. By itself, angioplasty is a fantastic procedure, and it enormously reduces chest pain and angina. However, the most dramatic and profound application of angioplasty is for treating the blocked coronary arteries that cause a heart attack. In this situation, the occluded coronary artery is unblocked with either balloons or with any of the new angioplasty devices, after which a heart stent is inserted. The stent reduces chances of recurrence of the blockage in the arteries and it provides a metallic scaffolding in the coronary artery.

Although I had performed several hundred Primary PCI procedures during my practice as an interventional cardiologist, this particular application of angioplasty was at best unscientific and relatively ineffective. By 2002, the leading cardiology societies, the American Heart Association and the American College of Cardiology societies added a critical directive to Primary PCI – a Door-to-Balloon (D2B) time was inserted into the guidelines. This was a seismic event in cardiology and this mandate has contributed to saving hundreds of thousands of lives. The new definition of D2B time was felt to be scientifically, medically, logistically, and legally prudent when treating occluded coronary arteries that were causing the heart attack. The D2B time converted the already pristine procedure of performing angioplasty for heart attacks. Primary PCI has achieved an iconic and life-saving status as a result of these mandates. Since every minute counts critically in opening the occluded artery to restore blood flow, a strict calculation of these performance times was required. This time was calculated from the moment the patient entered the door of the hospital to the time when the coronary artery was dilated – therein the origin of D2B time. It is important to understand some practical aspects of the D2B time.

For the patient, it meant that the occluded artery that was causing the heart attack would be urgently opened. Not when it was convenient for the doctor or for the hospital, but as a stringent medical (and medico-legal) requirement. Millions of patients have benefited as a result of this tough requirement. As opposed to the situation that existed previously when ad hoc primary angioplasty was performed for heart attacks, the new guideline mandated the obligation for the procedure to be performed urgently, nationwide, with strict D2B times. Logistically, the new mandates of performing urgent Primary PCI dramatically altered the specialty of Interventional Cardiology. For interventional cardiologists, such as me, who consented to provide Primary PCI and take a STEMI call, it was obligatory to reach the catheterization laboratory (cath lab, for short, the special room where angioplasty is performed in hospitals) within 30 minutes of being notified, twenty-four hours a day. This 30-minute response included driving time – and of course, the luck and skills to navigate traffic. It meant immediately abandoning whatever the cardiologist was engaged in, be that seeing patients in the office or at another hospital, or sleeping, or playing tennis. Every activity was terminated abruptly and the rush to the cath lab began. For the hospital, it meant the extra cost and logistics of keeping an on-call team available 24/7/365. During working hours, if the cath lab was busy and there was a patient with a heart attack, it meant taking off the elective patient off the operating table to permit the Primary PCI to be performed.

The nationwide adoption of urgent heart attack treatment with D2B times has been nothing short of revolutionary. It is disappointing that this fantastic feat performed by interventional cardiologists, nurses, technicians, ER staff and paramedics remains poorly acknowledged by society. Personnel performing this amazing procedure have largely remained unsung in their heroic saving of millions of lives.

Besides childbirth, I do not know of a more amazing procedure in medicine than Primary PCI, the amazing procedure that reliably and predictably aborts a heart attack. The entire "on call" heart attack team, at every hospital that performs PCI in the country has created protocols that enable this exercise in almost military fashion. At most hospitals, this team consists of two nurses, two technicians and the interventional cardiologists. All are activated with a single activation phone call and all must rush urgently to the cath lab.

Simultaneously, the ambulance services and paramedics act with coordinated urgency to diagnose, stabilize and transport this patient to the emergency room. Once in the hospital, the patient is immediately triaged and transported to the cath lab where primary angioplasty is performed. In expert hands, this procedure takes about 30 minutes, but it requires exceptional speed and skills.

Throughout this book, you will read about numerous such astonishing procedures, but the following should help you understand its true importance.

Imagine for a moment that your father is having a heart attack. The entire family is terrified of impending death of their loved one. Your mother is frightened that she will become a widow, and you are suddenly confronting a permanent loss of the person who gave you all. Your father is having profound chest pain, suffocating shortness of breath, extreme fear and anxiety, and he is losing consciousness as he is wheeled into the cath lab. About thirty minutes later, his vital signs have been restored, chest pain eliminated, his pallor and even his sense of humor is restored. A most devastating tragedy has now been averted. Not only has your father survived this calamitous heart attack, but also miraculously, there may be no damage to his heart muscle. In particular, if this procedure has been performed with short D2B time, that is often achieved from team work of the STEMI team.

Helping you, the reader, contribute to reducing the D2B time is the essence of "Planning for Your Heart Attack – and Surviving It." Allow me to explain.

We calculate the Door-to-Balloon time as the moment when the patient enters the hospital. Over the last 15 years, an army of experts has sacrificed enormously to reduce the Door-to-Balloon times. At almost every hospital, experts have deconstructed the STEMI chaos, all in an effort to save precious minutes to reduce D2B times. Remember, every minute counts when you are having a heart attack. At the hospital, we calculate the D2B time and use this as a scientific parameter to monitor our performance. The D2B times of the last decade have been reduced from 120 to 90 to 60 minutes. Each of this de- escalation of D2B times has required phenomenal improvement of performance at individual hospitals.

The D2B time is, however, controversial.

In truth, the real time that is critical begins from the moment the patient has chest pain. That is when the artery has often occluded and the heart attack has begun. Each minute of delay in opening the artery is resulting in death of the heart muscle. This is important to understand. Often the patient survives the heart attack but a portion of the heart muscle has been permanently scarred. If this damage is severe, the patient may experience fatigue, difficulty in breathing, and other symptoms that result from heart failure. The D2B time calculates the time from entering the hospital to having the artery open but it does not include the precious time that is lost before the patient reaches the hospital. Although a fast and well-trained team can dramatically reduce D2B times and the doctor can skillfully open the occluded artery, there may have been damage to the heart muscle from delays in reaching the hospital. Other system delays also cause the same end result. Irrespective, patient education is paramount to reduce precious time that is lost before reaching the hospital.

It is my intent to make this recognition of chest pain abundantly sharp for the reader. Sadly and tragically, an overwhelming majority of patients have had chest pain for hours before calling 9-1-1. Various psychological, emotional, social, financial, and personal barriers contribute to this delay. A fantastic and life-saving coordinated procedure by the entire team of paramedics, ER physicians, and interventional cardiologists is of no use for treating a patient who had been having chest pain for 6 hours before seeking help. In the ensuing chapters, I will make it pristinely clear how the bibliophile can identify these symptoms correctly and seek help for a life-preserving procedure. Sometimes, even the most brilliant professionals, as a result of fear and anxiety, miss these symptoms. I have performed primary angioplasty on 3 cardiologists who were making clinical runs, and who had failed to recognize their own heart attacks.

Therefore, the primary intent in "managing your heart attack" is for you, the reader, to identify symptoms of a heart attack and begin treatment immediately. Yourselves. Herein lies my greatest gift of life to the students of this book. Taking the time to prepare may be the best thing you will do in your life when confronted with a heart attack.

Let me reiterate the scientific fact again - every minute of delay in opening the artery results in permanent damage to the heart muscle. Therefore, the absolute mandate is performing this procedure immediately. Primary angioplasty not only saves your life, but also for the intelligent reader, who seeks immediate care, it prevents damage to the heart muscle that determines the quality of your life, and your symptom-free performance of life's activities. A delay in your recognition of heart attack hugely reduces the benefits of primary PCI. The heart team will still open the artery, but the damage may have been done. This book will make you an expert in eliminating this dreaded possibility that has remained my single biggest disappointment after performing, perhaps, the most primary angioplasties in the world. I have been dejected hundreds of times after urgently performing this procedure, only to recognize that I could not save the heart muscle because the patient presented late. Therein lies the purpose of writing this book – so that you, the patient, and I, the interventional cardiologist, can work together to not only open the artery that is causing the heart attack, but to preserve the heart muscle that you need for the rest of your life.

Not every chest pain causes a heart attack. This book will help you decipher if your chest discomfort is a result of a heart attack.

Let us now, understand one more, and possibly the last scientific fact as it relates to heart attacks.

Despite the remarkable procedure of primary angioplasty, I am only putting a Band- Aid to a systematic disease of atherosclerosis, the medical entity by which fat deposits in the arteries of the body. Primary angioplasty gets you out of the avalanche; the process of climbing the mountain to treat atherosclerosis is the next challenge. But primary angioplasty has now provided you the opportunity to get up and fight again. This is the second purpose of this book – to help you manage your risk factors through lifestyle modification. Often, after performing a primary angioplasty, I have meditated on how to prevent a further heart attack for that individual patient. The strategies that I will recommend to you for preventing a second heart attack have been collated from the meticulous conversations and observations from treating thousands of patients with heart attacks and understanding what they were doing wrong. There is a clear pattern of how heart attack occurs and very distinct modes of presentation. Unless the contributing factors are not urgently addressed, recurrence of the disease will happen. For various unfortunate reasons, our present healthcare delivery system rewards angioplasty and less so the mechanisms to prevent it. I have performed these amazing procedures for 15 years, and till this present moment, I have postponed bringing to the reader some simple measures that will prevent a second heart attack. I am determined to provide to you the wisdom gained from my experience. These lifestyle modifications will also help an individual to avoid a heart attack. Therefore, this dictum is equally important for a patient that has had a heart attack and for the one that is interested in avoiding one!

In essence, this book is continuing the fantastic success of life-saving D2B intervention and opening the dialogue with the patient about how to prevent further heart attacks.

Before I unfold these riddles, I want to share a few parts of this incredible journey that will help you understand the basis of my recommendations.

After performing more than 8,000 angioplasty procedures as an interventional cardiologist, I made a very conscious decision to dedicate my career to performing primary angioplasty. I understood, probably ahead of most cardiologists, the fantastic ways that a new specialty of a heart attack cardiologist could be created. For 15 years, I remain, perhaps, the world's only cardiologist, that performs primary angioplasty only. I have based some of these extremely difficult and strategic decisions on a most profound quotation from Mahatma Gandhi:

"In matters of conscience, the opinion of the majority does not count."

I threw away a thriving career as an interventional cardiologist and took up the extremely challenging task of performing primary angioplasty as a dedicated profession. Since every minute counted in performing this life-saving procedure, this systematically destroyed any semblance of a normal life that I had. I lost my sleep pattern, lived in surgical scrubs, was financially bankrupted, fought "traffic citations", survived accidents, and struggled for years in balancing a personal and a professional life. A majority of these procedures occur between midnight and 6 AM – to treat hearts attacks that are known to occur more often in the early morning hours. These personal sacrifices were hugely surpassed by the incredible gratification that comes from performing this dramatic procedure. Virtually every primary angioplasty saves a life. I have never taken for granted this amazing opportunity granted to me. To be able to save a life in 30 minutes through my immediate availability and complete focus is overwhelming to me, even after 15 years.

Spiritually, this, to me, is the sole reason for my existence. This was the larger purpose of my becoming a doctor and following the path of a great physician father.

In this journey, I first mastered the procedure. Performing a primary angioplasty at 10 a.m. and at 3 a.m. are totally different ball games. Instead of electively performing lucrative angioplasty, I ended up sleeping in dirty on-call rooms at hospitals. My own personal anxiety in living up to these demanding expectations caused me to have anxiety tremors in the initial years of this radical life change. I was on call 24 hours a day, anxiously anticipating the next call that would trigger instantaneous response.

Between 2004 and 2012, I averaged an astounding 252 nights on call each year. I proudly announce that in 15 years of performing this commission, it has never taken me more than 2 minutes to abandon whatever I was doing and jump into the car. Fortunately for millions of patients, I am not alone. Hundreds of cardiologists across the country and all over the world are responding to heart attacks in this precise manner. Where my intellect lies was in demonstrating an ability to advance heart attack angioplasty as a dedicated specialty.

After a few challenging months of beginning the life of a cardiologist dedicated to performing Primary PCI, it was obvious to me that this was a self-destroying lifestyle. But it was essential in my journey. Years later, as I taught this procedure to thousands of cardiologists worldwide, this experience was my earned capital. It remains so, to this day as I have continued to perform these procedures, now about 150 nights a year. This personal journey allowed me to implore cardiologists to work as hard, sacrifice sleep and rush to save lives. How could I expect other cardiologists to do the same without having lived in the trenches myself? It has often struck me, that till date, no cardiologist, anywhere, has protested to my calls to action for personal sacrifice to save patients' lives with Primary PCI. I attribute this, most of all, to practicing what I preach.

As years passed in this numbing exercise, it became abundantly clear to me that the larger task involved in primary PCI is not the "procedure" but the "process" of how a patient safely and quickly reaches the cath lab. Personally, this was the second chapter in my advance as a heart attack treating cardiologist.

For years, I had wondered why I had obtained a business degree in addition to being an interventional cardiologist. Suddenly and magically, this management experience came in extremely handy as I investigated improving efficiencies of the entire STEMI process. A quick explanation of this term, STEMI, which you will confront often in the remainder of the book, stands for ST-elevation myocardial infarction, the bigger and more intense presentation of a heart attack.

The new specialty I proposed was that of a STEMI cardiologist. This is a work in progress. I have become one of the first STEMI cardiologists and I have triggered a discussion whether this could be an entirely new discipline.

Returning to my own experience - my new assignments now

extended beyond performing the STEMI procedure. I was an earnest student trying to master the STEMI process. In pursuit of this knowledge, I began interacting with numerous EMS and ER experts. I understood the reasons that led to STEMI delay, and I methodically began to eliminate these obstacles. This task was much harder than the one of doing the procedure for which I had been trained and what was an extension of being an Interventional Cardiologist.

As my own progress continued, in the entire nation, the wheels of STEMI progress were turning. The EMS, including the ambulance and paramedics, became highly proficient in providing early care for heart attack patient. Intelligent ambulance coordination began at local EMS stations. Instead of the patient being taken to the nearest facility, legislative hurdles were eliminated so that patients could be taken directly to the nearest primary PCI hospital. Wireless transmission of EKG and pre-hospital activation of the STEMI team became a norm. Emergency Department or ED bypass, which enables the patient to be taken straight to the cath lab, began occurring for suitable patients. The entire nation's hospitals were now designated as either a STEMI facility or one that transported heart attack patients to one. Each STEMI institution now had an on-call team that responded urgently – this task is now seamlessly performed at more than 1,000 hospitals in our country. It is the sacrifice of these dedicated professionals that has extended the amazing primary angioplasty procedure to millions of patients with heart attacks.

I created a dedicated Heart Attack Symposium, Lumen, in Miami to teach the lessons I had learned to perform Primary PCI. Ten years after conducting this meeting in Miami, I converted it to Lumen Global. Today, Lumen Global is one of the world's premier heart attack conventions and it is rotated through major metropolitan capitals. My SINCERE database has led to numerous peer-reviewed publications, and it has yielded 5 textbooks.

The philanthropic Lumen Foundation, which I founded in 2006, is now assisting more than 30 developing countries with education, training, and research about heart attacks and for creating STEMI networks. In the last few years, we have utilized telemedicine to facilitate heart attack management for poor patients in Brazil and Colombia. My most recent research endeavor is to identify and reduce barriers that prevent women in seeking access to heart attack treatment in developing countries.

I am delighted that my aspiration to educate the amateur about this journey has now being fulfilled.

I sincerely hope that the following chapters will contribute to saving lives from heart attacks – beginning with yours!

...AND SURVIVING IT

CHAPTER 1. CARLOS

Kites rise highest against the wind - not with it.
Winston Churchill

Flat line. (Cardiac arrest).
Shock. (Deliver electric shock to the heart to revive the patient).
No response.
Shock again.
Feel the pulse. Check for the rhythm. Continue CPR. Give another dose of epinephrine. Check the bicarb. Shock again. (This is the routine checklist of drugs and resuscitation techniques to keep the vital organs alive during a CPR).
Wait... wait. We have a rhythm. Stop CPR.
"Feel the pulse... Good. Check the blood pressure.
"Doctor, v-fib again." (The most malignant heart rhythm, if not immediately converted to a more stable rhythm, this is fatal very quickly).
Shock, 360 J. (The electrical energy required for converting the malignant rhythm).
No pulse, no blood pressure. Flat line. Continue CPR.
Shock again. Bicarb. Calcium.
V-fib again. Shock. "We have a pulse." Blood pressure is 100, signs.
"Get an EKG stat... 8mm ST segment elevation in leads 2,3, AVF." (EKG changes suggesting a heart attack).
Meet Carlos Cruz! This was supposed to be another routine day in the life of this 48-year-old construction worker. Carlos woke up at his usual 7 AM. His wife, Miranda, had already got their daughter, Anna, ready for school. Anna was bubbling with excitement, as it was her 7th birthday. Instead of Miranda dropping Anna off at school, on this special day, both Carlos and Miranda got into their Chrysler van and drove their cheerful daughter to Coral Gables Elementary. Then, both enjoyed a tranquil breakfast at I Hop next to Coral Gables Elementary School.
Living had been hard, but now both Miranda and Carlos had stable and well- paying jobs, and they had moved into their new apartment in Coconut Grove.
Life was finally looking up.
Carlos began work at the construction site in his supervisory role at the new I-826 ramp extension. A few hours later, after his routine lunch,

something did not seem right. He had a strange heaviness in the chest as he walked up the ramp to monitor the pouring of the concrete. There was clear discomfort now. He raised his left hand to his chest and rubbed gently. At this precise moment, he crashed to the ground and became unconscious. Fortunately, the workers had witnessed his fall. One of them immediately called 9-1-1.

Carlos recovered quickly. He sat up, completely dazed. "I am going to die. Help me," he fumbled.

As John, the site engineer, bent down to speak to Carlos, he noticed him to be completely pale and sweating. Carlos was disoriented. He now complained of excruciating chest pain. He clutched his chest and fainted again.

Armando and Heidi were the paramedics who responded to the EMS. In precisely, 6 minutes and 34 seconds, their ambulance had reached Carlos, whom they found unconscious and in ventricular fibrillation. He was immediately shocked and he again regained consciousness. He was quickly placed on the stretcher and urgently rushed to Bayside Medical Center, 0.7 miles away.

This was going to be a day that Carlos, Miranda, and Anna would remember forever.

For Dr. Franco, the ER physician at Bayside Medical Center, the diagnosis was upfront STEMI. The hospital protocol instructed immediate primary angioplasty. Dr. Franco yelled to Nancy, the unit secretary, to call code STEMI. Instantaneously, the hospital operator announced twice, "Code STEMI, Code STEMI."

With this coordinated and single phone call, the operator activated the entire STEMI team on call.

It was 2:11 PM. The on-call team of nurses, Phillip and Brenda, responded immediately. Jack Herrera and Orlando Garcia were the technicians, and both sprung immediately, almost in military fashion, to their assigned STEMI duties. Orlando turned on the X Ray equipment and the computer systems that would be required for the emergency procedures. Jack quickly opened the surgical kit and he began connecting the numerous tubes that would deliver the drugs and that were required to monitor the patient's blood pressure and heart rhythm. The nurses, Phillip and Brenda rushed to the emergency room to transport the STEMI patient.

The team had dealt with such situations before and they went about their urgent tasks with practiced ease.

However, something was amiss.

Dr. Baker, the interventional cardiologist, was scrubbed in another angioplasty procedure at Baptist Hospital, almost 30 minutes away. A few urgent calls were required to track him down.

Dr. Baker answered and informed that he was unable to respond immediately to this dire emergency.

Back to Carlos, who had again developed asystole (cardiac arrest).

CPR with vigorous chest compression was reinitiated; an anesthesiologist rapidly inserted a breathing tube.

Carlos was now on life support. Precious minutes were ticking before irreversible brain damage would set in.

CPR was continued as per the protocol. The "Code Team" of eight, including doctors, nurses, and technicians, were frantically performing several simultaneous maneuvers to keep Carlos alive.

Miranda, Carlos's wife, had received a call from John, the site engineer. Her friend, Jenny, had driven her to the ER. She was inconsolable and in panic. She needed to be calmed and comforted by the ER staff. "Save my husband. Save Carlos," she uttered incoherently. She searched shakily for her brother's phone number, dialed him amidst this mad confusion, and asked him to rush to the hospital. She had hung up the phone, and now her brother was calling to ask, "which hospital?" In this chaos, she told her brother that Carlos had "a massive heart attack" and "Carlos is going to die." She had asked her brother to come to the ER, and then hung up the phone without mentioning it was at Bayside Medical Center!

Carlos was now intubated and CPR was ongoing. The EKG demonstrated a massive heart attack. But, Dr. Baker, the on-call cardiologist, was not available.

Dr. Franco now considered using TNK, the clot-buster drug, for treating the heart attack. However, he was concerned about the prolonged CPR that could create complications with TNK. "Is there no other interventional cardiologist around?" he yelled? "Please find someone."

I was picking ripe mangoes in our backyard when my cell phone rang. This was not unusual. I had previously responded on numerous occasions to bail out for heart attack patients. Fortunately, I lived across the street from the hospital, and it had become famously known at Bayside Medical Center that Dr. Mehta could be reached at all times. To demonstrate my belief in STEMI interventions in the early formative years, I had deliberately made my availability known to the staff.

Immediately upon hearing about this critical patient, I informed the ER that I would be on the way and ordered to continue CPR.

In about 3 minutes, already in scrubs, I dashed into the ER. As I sprinted across, I vividly remember glancing through the corner of my eyes, a wailing woman - Miranda.

It had now been 26 minutes of CPR and the patient had been shocked 15 minutes. Dr. Franco was about to pronounce Carlos dead!

Ordinarily, I would have agreed with him. But this situation was clearly different. Carlos had a witnessed cardiac arrest; CPR had been begun immediately and a very skilled team had performed it uninterruptedly. The EKG demonstrated a clear and massive heart attack. We simply could not let Carlos die.

I took over Carlos' charge, and to Dr. Franco's supreme credit, he relinquished care immediately. My cath lab team was already there and the lab was ready.

The EKG showed a massive inferior wall myocardial infarction. I immediately surmised the culprit to be an occluded Right Coronary artery (one of the two major arteries that supply the heart muscle).

A house physician, Dr. Nader, was performing CPR with robust chest compressions. He had been alternating with Ralph, one of the respiratory technicians, who had just stepped off after about 5 minutes of performing intense CPR. Ralph was sweating profusely.

I quickly asked Ralph and Dr. Nader if they could continue CPR as we wheeled the patient to the cath lab. Both emphatically agreed. The proficient ER nurses disconnected all lines and electrical connections, and we were ready to wheel. A security guard sprinted ahead and quickly secured the elevator. Dr. Nader balanced himself on the moving stretcher by planning his feet on the bottom bars and continued chest compressions. The team reconfigured as the patient was wheeled into the elevators. The defibrillator was placed between the patient's feet and Brenda maintained a cautious look at the heart rhythm. The respiratory technicians monitored the mechanical ventilator and Dr. Nader was doing CPR.

Saving a patient's life from a heart attack with a STEMI intervention is a practiced art with intense training and teamwork. Almost always, the success is attributed to the Interventional Cardiologist. I can attest to the fact that the nurses and technicians who assist the procedure, as was evident in the care of Carlos, are the unsung heroes of a STEMI intervention. It is their supreme dedication and sacrifice, often in very trying circumstances that contribute to saving patient lives with Primary PCI.

We made it safely in the delicate elevator ride – although just three floors needed to be climbed, with all the equipment and precise ventilation and chest compression, this was a highly proficient task. The team had most admirably performed it.

However, just as we exited the elevator and as we were outside the cath lab, Carlos' heart again went into malignant ventricular fibrillation.
"V. Fib," yelled Brenda.

Everyone stepped off and away from the stretcher so as not to get the electric shock (routine protocol to prevent electric shock).

Carlos' chest was delivered another thumping 360 joules current. Again, his body was thrust up with the sheer magnitude of the electric shock. However, it immediately converted his heart rhythm to normal.

We continue to proceed into the room.

Once again, the ugly rhythm returned and once again it was restored by a perfectly coordinated counter shock. The regression to the ugly rhythm was relentless.

We pressed on. Carlos was now on the cath lab table and we had a shot to begin the urgent procedure. The intensive care specialist, or as we call it, the intensivist, Dr. Nathan, had now joined us and he took charge of the CPR, as I dashed out to scrub and put on my lead suit. This equipment is needed to protect the operator from X Rays.

Ralph continued chest compressions most expertly, pausing for a moment to permit the quick covering of the patient's body with surgical scrubs. Both he and Dr. Nader had quickly put on lead suits, as did the technicians that were handling the ventilator. Jack, the cath lab technician expertly prepped both groins for the procedure. Brenda tied my surgical gown and helped me with surgical gloves, Phillip checked the intravenous lines and began documenting on his cath procedure log sheet. I was ready to stick the groin with the surgical needle.

I felt no pulses in the right or left femoral arteries. This made the task more challenging. I proceeded to use the anatomy landmarks to locate the blood vessel and injected local anesthetic to numb the area. I was fortunate to penetrate the Right Femoral artery with the first stick. This artery would provide access to reach the heart and the coronary arteries.

With a routinely used JR4 catheter, I was immediately able to introduce it in the Right Coronary Artery. I had suspected this to be the culprit vessel based upon the EKG. This particular conclusion is fairly easy and cardiologists can easily predict which of the three major coronary arteries would be blocked (there are two coronary arteries, left and right but the left gives rise to two major branches, making it a total of three large coronary arteries).

The trick was balancing the equipment with the ongoing CPR. Both the technician Orlando and I kept repositioning the catheters and the other plastic manifold that connects multiple intravenous drips and the iodine-based dye that is injected via a hand held syringe.

As I manipulated the equipment, I periodically shouted out to Dr. Nader to hold compression. We both coordinated our activities in this fashion over the next few minutes of critical activity. I needed Dr. Nader to pause to enable me to do the critical and fine movements of catheters and wires in the heart. Dr. Nader's fine job of pumping the chest enabled blood to perfuse the brain and other vital organs. Brenda was ready to pounce the chest if the heart rhythm degenerated.

As Dr. Nader paused again upon my command, in one coordinated movement, I operated the cath lab table with the left hand and injected 3-4 cc of radiocontrast agent into the catheter with my left hand.

The Right Coronary Artery was 100% blocked. The culprit had

been identified. Could I now open this occluded artery fast? Would this result in restoring the heart rhythm and function? Could it save Carlos?

At my direction, Brenda injected Angiomax, a drug that prevents formation of blood clots on the catheters and wires that I was using. I then quickly took a standard guide   wire that I was going to use to cross the blocked Right Coronary Artery.

But, Carlos' heart was motionless. That had been evident under X Rays. Would the angioplasty revive it?

Were we simply pushing our luck? Was I being unrealistic? Was my faith that   we would be able to save Carlos ill founded? Were we simply too late in attempting these heroics? Would brain damage not have occurred?

There was no time to reflect. We must press on. A life was at stake. No effort was too much. Continue with everything – CPR, angioplasty! We can succeed. Still.

Dr. Nader had switched with Ralph. He paused with the chest compressions as I steered the guide wire across the occluded Right Coronary Artery under X-Ray guidance. Ralph's incredible dedication and skill was evident when he rapidly thrust a quick series of chest compressions before pausing to permit me to go back on X Rays.

I have often wondered about this remarkable procedure and about the contributions of Dr. Nader and Ralph. It has left me mesmerized. Their dedication was commendable. Both were selfless and uncaring for their own wellbeing in their heroic efforts. As they performed CPR, they ended up being close to the source of radiation. Irrespective, both stuck to their life-saving task.

The occluded Right Coronary artery was not difficult to cross with the guide wire. I easily navigated it beyond the blockage. I now needed to quickly inflate and deflate a balloon catheter at the precise site of the blockage to create an opening for blood to pass forward and on to the heart muscle.

Brenda had opened the balloon catheter that I had asked for. She handed it to Orlando who expertly prepared it in a flash. Ralph released another quick series of compressions before pausing again.

With my foot, I again activated the X Rays and quickly positioned the balloon at the site of occlusion. Then, yelled to Orlando to dilate the balloon with the pressure gauge. Expertly, Orlando dialed up the inflation device that dilated the balloon catheter. We deflated after 10 seconds and I quickly injected the dye to see if we had created an opening.

What followed was nothing short of a miracle. As dramatic as anything I had witnessed in my career. The fruit of our labor, the magnificent result of angioplasty to treat heart attacks. The artery was widely patent and there was a brisk flow of blood that rushed to feed the heart muscle. The rhythm restored to normal, the blood pressure came up instantaneously. I placed a stent, the tiny steel scaffold that maintains the patency of the vessel. It was routine and simple, now that Carlos's heart was pumping vigorously. CPR was discontinued and the gallant team that had worked so hard left to go back to their regular duties. Their fantastic work had saved Carlos.

The magic of Primary Angioplasty was there for all to see, and for Carlos to experience! Beginning from that precise moment when the blocked vessel was dilated till Carlos left the hospital, his heart did not have a single extra beat.

I continued to complete the procedure. The Left Coronary artery did not have any blockage. I then infused a small amount of dye into the left ventricle, the pumping chamber of the heart to check its function. The left ventricle was completely normal. There was no dead or scarred heart muscle.

All this was happening in a patient who was about to be pronounced dead just a few minutes ago!

After a heart attack, the patient's fate largely depends on the heart muscle. This subject is extremely important for you to understand. When you comprehend these facts, it will become very clear why it is imperative to treat heart attacks urgently. And why you must seek care immediately.

Miraculously, Carlos's heart muscle did not suffer damage. This was on account of the artery being opened very quickly despite the very deadly way in which the heart attack presented. Of course, Carlos was very lucky too. He was relatively young and there was no previous heart disease. After a heart attack, if the heart muscle is normal, the patient can expect a normal and healthy life without much restriction. However, if there is damage to the heart muscle, there can be debilitating symptoms. Physical activity can be limited and there is a need for numerous drugs to maintain adequate pumping of the heart.

Many of the patients that are seen in cardiologist's office for fatigue and difficulty in breathing had their heart muscle damaged previously from a heart attack. If this damage is severe, it can result in heart failure which is a very serious condition that requires very careful treatment.

The damage to the heart muscle may have occurred from their heart attack not having been treated and the heart muscle dying from the lack of blood supply from the blocked artery. Sometimes, the damage results despite the artery being opened with angioplasty or with clot buster drugs. Often, this occurs from there being delay in the treatment. In such cases, although their arteries were dilated, the heart muscle had sustained damage. Many of these patients' experience life-long and debilitating symptoms of heart failure. It is these unfortunate patients that may require placement of complex, expensive and complicated heart devices such as heart pacemakers and implanted defibrillators to treat their heart failure. Infrequently, these patients will be candidates for heart transplant. Hospital readmissions may be frequently required for treating exacerbations of the heart failure. The quality of life is severely limited. Death may also occur within a few years of sustaining severe heart failure. Healthcare costs for treating heart failure run in billions and the impact on the patient, the family and to society is enormous.

Herein is the enlightening message of this book – delay in recognizing the symptoms of a heart attack can result in permanent heart damage and life-long symptoms of heart failure. Delay in seeking care and system delays in providing the treatment have the same effect. Every minute is precious for a patient having a heart attack. Immediately recognizing the heart attack and calling for help is critical. A coordinated and well-trained ambulance service and expert paramedics are vital for your survival, both to save your life and to prevent the permanent damage to your heart muscle. Reaching the right hospital that performs Primary PCI is central to your survival. Having a skilled cardiologist do this procedure is paramount. Having a well-trained team is an absolute essential.

By reading about Carlos, you will understand how each of these steps contributed to saving has life.

How does a person know these complex matters? This information is not readily available. I have not seen public education campaigns teaching patients about these matters. You cannot expect to be searching Google when you are having a heart attack. Your heart attack will not announce itself. You need to be prepared. This book will provide you with this information and with knowledge to navigate you easily through this haze.

Indeed, our country has created fantastic institutions to treat heart attacks with an army of trained personnel and with the availability of expensive equipment. These are lacking in most parts of the world. We must recognize how fortunate we are and we must intelligently use these services. Unfortunately, all these resources are of no use, unless the patient recognizes the symptoms and seeks immediate help.

Read on – soon, you will become an expert in identifying a heart attack, and in doing so, you will "Prepare for your Heart Attack … and survive it" by assimilating the simple advice that is presented in future chapters of the book.

To continue the most amazing survival story of Carlos, he was extubated effortlessly the same evening, he was joking by dinnertime and walking the next morning. Carlos left the hospital with a broad grin on his face on the third day of his hospitalization for a cardiac arrest and acute myocardial infarction. The look in Miranda's eyes said it all – relief, gratitude, prayers, for doctors that performed this amazing procedure that saved her husband's life.

To capture the statistics – from the moment the EMS wheeled in Carlos post-cardiac arrest to my opening the occluded right Coronary Artery took us 84 minutes. From the time of my administering the local anesthetic to re-canalizing the artery was a mere 6 minutes.

Carlos' story is the story of Primary PCI, of the raging success of American Cardiology. It has made available to all Americans the tremendous benefits of this fantastic procedure.

On days when I am exhausted after treating several patients with their heart attacks, I remember Carlos, Miranda and Ana, and how this procedure saved not only Carlos, but also the entire family.

CHAPTER 2. THE ACCOUNTANT

It may be the cock that crows, but it is the hen that lays the eggs.
Margaret Thatcher

Grace was already up. It was 5:15 in the morning. She had taken a shower and had come downstairs to finish packing for their fantastic trip that morning. Victor, her husband, a baseball fanatic, was going to watch the Marlins play the Reds in Cincinnati that afternoon. Grace and Victor had planned this trip with their friends Rita and Mark Cruz. Mark was a Hall-of-Famer, retired baseball professional, and the families had known each other since 1974. It was going to be a terrific trip.

Perhaps not...

Victor came downstairs in his pajamas and announced, "I don't feel well." Grace inquired what was happening. She looked at him and she was immediately concerned. Victor looked pale. Rubbing his chest, Victor pointed to the center of it and said, "I am having chest pain."

"It must be your reflux," Grace said, referring to the long-standing stomach problem that Victor had.

"I don't think so." Victor replied, "I already took the Gaviscon, and it did not help. This seems very different."

Grace's father, who had passed away two years ago, was a noted ENT surgeon. Grace remembered many lessons that she had learned while observing her father. These were going to come in extremely helpful that morning.

She rushed to the medicine cabinet and grabbed the aspirin and nitroglycerin bottles, as well as the blood pressure kit. She first gave four tablets of aspirin and told Victor to swallow them. She then checked his blood pressure. It was 130/80; that seemed okay. But Victor had visibly worsened. He was extremely pale and sweating profusely.

Grace told Victor, "You are having a heart attack."

I want to alert the reader that the mysteries of heart attack will begin unfolding from this chapter onwards. This incident occurred on September 17, 2009, almost 7 years ago. To authenticate these events, I just had a long conversation with Grace. My memory about this incident has somewhat faded – the angioplasty procedure, I remember clearly. But the events leading to it that hold the important message for you, are less sharp in my mind. In my SINCERE database of all heart attack patients that I have ever treated, is a "remarks" column, where I meticulously note down

10

unique features of some cases. In Victor's column is scribbled "role of patient education." To most effectively recommend these precise teaching points, I embarked, as stated above, to speak to Grace.

Grace's father, the ENT surgeon, had written a prescription of nitroglycerin for Grace. Call it a father's love for a child, or some premonition. Irrespective, Grace had filled the nitroglycerin prescription, and she even knew how to administer it properly. She placed a nitroglycerin tablet under Victor's tongue and rushed to call 9-1-1.

Grace told the operators, "My husband is having a heart attack."

She had a brief conversation of about 40 seconds with the operators, and the ambulance, truck number 14, reached her within 5 minutes.

How fortunate are we in the United States! Think of what would happen to you if you lived in some other part of the world.

In my lectures about heart attack management in numerous countries, I pronounce, "your fate with a heart attack depends on your zip code." I explain further in this manner. If your zip code is 10023 (our second home in NYC), were you to have a heart attack there, the following will be the likely scenario. An ambulance would reach your door within 5 to 7 minutes. You will be transported to a PCI institution and have a short Door- to-Balloon STEMI intervention of about 60 minutes. You will probably not have damage to your heart muscle. Furthermore, you will be discharged from the hospital on the third day on a few simple medications. The chances of your dying from this heart attack would be less than 2% (a decade ago, this number was about 6%). It is also entirely possible that you would probably forget that this incident ever happened. You would continue to have an unhampered physical life because of speedy and expert management of your heart attack.

Now imagine your zip code to be 110026, the home where I grew up in New Delhi, India. The following unfortunate scenario is likely to unfold in this situation.

It will highlight the statement I made above about our being incredibly fortunate with good healthcare in the United States. It is a blessing that we take for granted. The enormous reduction in death rates from heart attacks has contributed to our improving life expectancy. If you have significantly reduced the possibly of death from the single biggest cause of death – heart attacks, then it clearly impacts how long you will live. Several recent studies have revealed what some cardiologists have already experienced – the dramatic improvements with Primary PCI in the United States have significantly reduced the death rate from heart disease. In "A Sea Change in Treating Heart Attacks," (June 19, 2015, The New York Times), Gina Kollta reports that the death rate from coronary heart disease has dropped 30% in a decade, and the reason for that is that hospitals, rich and poor, have streamlined emergency treatment. She further writes that heart attacks are no longer the biggest cause of death.

The New York Times report, while heartening, must not ring in complacency for either doctors or patients. That would be unfortunate. There are numerous additional areas of further improvement that I will highlight in the book. We can do better still and further perfect how heart attacks are being managed. This prudence notwithstanding, a nationwide availability of Primary PCI is a seismic event. It is life changing for thousands of patients. These developments are uplifting – the biggest killer of men and women in the United States may no longer be heart attacks. This is truly a fantastic medical achievement that is a result of dedicated paramedics, ED/ER physicians, cardiologists, nurses and technicians. This feat should be celebrated as a national triumph.

Back to the destiny of a heart attack patient in the heart of New Delhi. There is at least a 30% chance that a patient with heart attack in zip code 110026 will never reach a hospital. Death would probably occur from the complications of a heart attack. Mostly, these include a severe heart blockage that interrupts the coordinated pumping of the heart chambers or a malignant rhythm disorder known as ventricular fibrillation (remember Carlos). The third dreaded complication occurs when the lungs backlog with blood that cannot be pumped forward by the failing heart. In all probability, the patient with a heart attack in New Delhi would reach the hospital himself. This happens in almost 96% of the cases and it is very unfortunate. Self-transportation is the overwhelmingly common means of reaching a hospital for patients that are suffering a heart attack. It is most likely that this hospital would have no availability of expert heart attack management, let alone providing primary angioplasty. In some cases, a richer patient is able to access a better-equipped private hospital where excellent care is possible. But for the majority of the patients, this service is not available. Most likely, the smaller hospital would treat the heart attack with an older (and less expensive) clot buster drug. The chances of dying from such a heart attack in the zip code 110026 may be as high as 8-10%, several times higher than for a heart attack in zip code 10023. Worse, there is also a strong possibility of permanent damage to the heart muscle. As I discussed in the previous chapter, this damage to the heart muscle causes lifelong limitation of physical activity.

Getting back to Victor and Grace, the paramedics speedily performed a 12- lead EKG, the standard way of diagnosing numerous heart attacks and several other heart disorders. As the name implies, 12 electrodes are placed across the arms, the legs, and on the chest to perform this 12-lead EKG. Trained technicians can accomplish this entire procedure in about 2 minutes. It can be easily done with a portable machine. The result is a long paper strip of EKG tracing from which numerous heart conditions, such as heart rhythm disorders, heart attacks and electrolyte imbalances, can be diagnosed. The most prodigious application for the EKG is for diagnosing heart attacks.

The EKG is an extremely simple test to perform. The equipment is relatively inexpensive and portable, and it is available in the smallest clinics and in doctors' offices. The technician obtaining an EKG simply has to learn a few anatomical landmarks where the 12 leads need to be placed. The machine performs a calibration that occurs on a special paper that has 1mm squares imprinted to enable calculation of time intervals. Our amazing heart generates electrical impulses and waveforms that are luminously captured in the EKG. This test, invented in 1860 by the brilliant Nobel laureate, Willem Einthoven, is a fundamental test of heart function.

Almost all of us, at some time in our lives, have had an EKG. We may even remember our doctor telling us to keep a copy of the EKG safely. This is more difficult to do than said, as the tracings fade over time. Therefore, if you have an EKG, make a digital copy of it. The purpose of archiving the EKG is simple; it is to compare with subsequent EKGs. Often it is not the changes in the present EKG, but comparisons with the past EKG that determines the significance of the new changes.

A most instructive part of heart attack management is that a heart attack can be diagnosed with a simple, easily performed, and readily available, EKG. This amazing test reliably diagnoses heart attacks – accuracy, in expert hands, can reach 95-98%.

How many medical entities do we know where such accuracy can be achieved with a single and simple investigation? Think of the numerous hospital and doctor visits, the multitude of X-rays, CT's, MRI's, nuclear scans, blood tests, and other investigations, that are often required for diagnosing various diseases. It is this particular novelty, of the simplicity and ease of diagnosing heart attacks with a simple EKG that is almost unique in medicine. Telemedicine, the remote guidance by an expert, is very powerful for managing heart attacks, for this precise reason. The expert diagnoses the heart attack from a remote location by his interpretation of the EKG that is easily transmitted to him.

The ease of performing the EKG is counterbalanced by the knowledge of the person interpreting it. There are several medical conditions in which the EKG tracings mimic a heart attack. In medicine, we call this a differential diagnosis. The process of narrowing down a differential diagnosis to an accurate diagnosis includes analysis of the patient's clinical history, presentation and the investigation. The accuracy of the EKG is therefore enhanced by the patient's clinical presentation. This clinical presentation is very diverse. Heart attacks present in a very different manner in men and in women. The elderly may not have classical symptoms of a heart attack at all. Diabetics, that comprise a large proportion of patients with heart attacks, often do not have chest pain. These perplexing clinical presentations can be missed both by patients and doctors.

In the illustrated cases that I have selected for this book, it will be my effort to present actual patients that may remind you of yourself and of your loved one, including, and most critically, your parents and grandparents. Through these sample patients, you will get a fairly accurate assessment of whether you are confronting a heart attack. A missed heart attack and a wrong diagnosis of chest pain is one of the most common medical errors. Chest pain can originate from diseases of the alimentary canal, mainly its upper portions that includes the food pipe, or the esophagus, and from the stomach. The erosive stomach acids mimic chest pain from a heart attack. Presentations can be so blindingly similar that it may be extremely difficult to differentiate the two.

This was happening with "The Accountant" who had a previous history of reflux disease. To relieve this, as he did during previous times, he took Gaviscon. In reflux disease, the acids from the stomach regurgitate back into the food pipe, or the esophagus, causing a sensation of burning or pain. This is not unlike what happens in chest pain from a heart attack. What differentiates the two is the presence of coronary risk factors or the predisposing conditions that make a patient more prone to heart attacks. A discussion and a profound understanding of these contributing risk factors and their management is the foundational pillars of this book. It will be addressed in detail in "The Accountant" and in numerous other parts of this book.

I would like to probe further into the EKG and its relevance to heart attack management. As the nation made progress in creating heart attack management systems, we focused on the absolute mandate of doing an EKG in patients presenting with chest pain. The immediate prerequisite to perform an EKG is the principle that guides "chest pain centers," advertised in the large hoardings you find on highways. Every patient with chest pain should immediately have a 12-lead EKG performed. This dramatically narrows the differential diagnosis of chest pain. It is now a system-wide recommendation in our country that any patient who presents with chest pain to any emergency room should have an EKG performed within 5 minutes of presentation. This has become standard practice and it has contributed to saving thousands of lives.

The pathway of obtaining EKGs in an ambulance is more complicated. Who should interpret this EKG? There are two broad ways of handling this in order to maximize diagnostic accuracy. We can either train the paramedics to become experts in reading EKGs, as has been successfully done by Dr. Michel Le May in Ottawa, Canada. Dr. Le May's advanced paramedics undergo rigorous training and they have been known to interpret EKGs with the same accuracy as cardiologists. However, this is difficult and expensive to do in our country with its large population. An alternative, which has been practiced in the United States and in several other countries, is to employ technology to assist us in more accurately diagnosing the EKG. With this method, an EKG is either wirelessly transmitted or faxed from the ambulance to the emergency room where the doctor is able to physically look at the tracings. Often, a second transmission of the EKG occurs between the ER and the cardiologist on STEMI call. A major initiative is underway in our country to place wireless technology in ambulances for transmitting the EKG.

The role of innovations, such as WhatsApp, cannot be overstated, when used for the purpose of transmitting the EKG. However, there is an important caveat to this easy mechanism – patient confidentiality that must be safeguarded with open access systems.

So, as taxpayers, it should be your burden to decree that the fire rescue ambulance in your tax district be equipped with EKG transmission capability. Doing so, you put your tax dollars into saving your life in case of a heart attack. Therefore, to increase your chance of surviving a heart attack, or" preparing for a heart attack," here is a two- part public mandate that you should petition for. 1) The ambulance transporting a heart attack patient should have a proven pathway to transmit EKG. 2) A heart attack patient must be transported to a primary PCI center rather than to the nearest hospital.

You will note how these features contributed to saving the life of the Accountant. Here are further observations about our solid healthcare system as it compares to several other countries.

A disclosure is needed at this stage. As I wrote the above paragraph, I changed "fantastic" to "solid" healthcare system. I even searched for less complimentary terms. There are clear deficiencies in our healthcare system. Noticeably, it fails the test of providing universal coverage. Beyond that, the major problem with our healthcare system is the extreme high cost of healthcare. It is cost-ineffective. Prohibitively so. I personally attribute much of this enormous expense to waste, fraud and to the unchecked costs of drugs and devices. In 1998, I completed a Masters in Business Management with a specialization in healthcare. I have alluded in different sections how the education in logistical management has contributed to my ability to create efficient heart attack processes and programs in various countries. To my academic education about healthcare was added a personal experience of watching healthcare in dozens of countries around the world.

The "solid" healthcare downgraded from "fantastic" is a result of this background.

As it relates to heart attack management, I emphatically believe that an efficient and reliable ambulance system is the key to saving lives from heart attacks. You must get involved in your community to demand excellent ambulance care. In almost every case that I have cited in the book, you will immediately recognize the contribution of the paramedics in saving lives. An excellent ambulance system with well-trained paramedics is one of the most distinguishing features of a progressive society. Think back about how much time you spent in learning about schools in the community where you wanted to move. We also know how home prices are higher in better school districts. But have you paused to learn about your ambulance system? Are they not equally important? We have no rating system for our ambulance system and for the paramedics. Of course, there is considerable variation in our ambulance systems. This is a field that has largely stayed beyond the public domain. Performance of STEMI at individual hospitals has not been ranked. These are new concepts. But are they not essential? Your outcome with the entity that has the highest likelihood of killing you depends on the caliber of your ambulance system. It also depends upon legislative unblocking that is required for EMS to transport the heart attack patient to the Primary PCI hospital directly. It also depends directly on the individual performance of the STEMI team at the Primary PCI hospital. Not to mention, on the expertise of the Interventional Cardiologist.

So, yes, most of us can rattle the statistics about the public school in our taxing district, but critical aspects that may save us from heart attacks, have never been discussed. I hope that I have steered you on with these poignant queries about the care that may be available in your community for heart attacks. These are novel thoughts and as a progressive society, it should behoove us to research these important matters and remain proactive. There is a strong scientific basis for these deliberations. The time to act is now!

Allow me to explain. A colleague who graduated with me in India wrote to me a few months after my 12th Annual Lumen Global symposium in New Delhi, India. It was a long email, the relevant sentence is, "now I fully understand your message at the meeting and what you kept emphasizing about saving lives from heart attacks." He had just lost his beloved brother from an ill-managed heart attack!

It is time for you to explore specifics about ambulance care in your community and details about the STEMI program at your local hospital. These queries are bound to improve the services.

On the topic of ambulance systems, our ambulance system is nowhere near the best in the world. Scandinavian countries, France, and even the UK, may have better ambulance services. However, this comparison is unscientific as it is much easier to provide intelligent ambulance systems in small countries. I have, however, been appalled to see the meager ambulance services in various, so-called advanced countries. They are unable to perform EKG and they lack telemetry, the ability to do continuous monitoring of the heart rhythm, an absolute essential capability when transporting a patient with a heart attack. In some other parts of the world, ambulances are merely "medical taxis". Even in providing this service, they often have a conflict of interest in taking paying patients to hospitals that have funded their operations. Another distressing phenomenon with ambulance service is seen in several hospitals in Asia, Africa, and in South America - ambulances are owned by individual hospitals. With this structure, patients directly call the hospital that dispatches its own ambulance to bring them to the hospital. This can often be extremely effective considering the lack of centralized ambulance services. Some hospitals are even able to send a doctor with the ambulance, and this is absolutely fantastic. However, this system is impractical as such ambulances make a two-way journey, often in heavy traffic, once to pick up the patient, and once to transport the patient to the hospital.

It is my experience with so many deficiencies, that I rated our healthcare solid. I also believe that by and large, the United States has an excellent ambulance structure with very well-trained paramedics.

An intelligent, centralized ambulance system is an absolute requirement of heart attack systems. In my lectures about heart attack treatment, in numerous countries, I have emphasized the need for improving ambulance systems. I have even gone to the extent of calling an ambulance, "the heart attack management center."

Treatment of a patient with a heart attack must begin in the ambulance, and possibly in the home, as demonstrated by Grace in treating "The Accountant.

In an ambulance, a heart attack can be diagnosed, the EKG transmitted, the patient stabilized, deadly complications managed, medications begun and the patient educated. Do you not deserve to know that this is occurring in your community?

As a nation, we must continue to invest more in improving the availability and performance of our ambulance systems. We must also invest in training and retraining of our paramedics. By doing so, we would dramatically improve our healthcare delivery. Specifically, in addition to heart attack management, this enormously assists in the management of strokes, which has numerous parallels with the urgent treatment of heart attacks.

The digression from Victor and Grace was a necessary exercise in educating you about managing your own situation. Let us return to Victor, the accountant. The paramedics have just performed the EKG.

It shows what Grace had observed right away – Victor was having a massive heart attack!

In medical terms, this was a myocardial infarction, the scientific term for a heart attack. It implies damage and necrosis of heart muscle as a result of occlusion of one of the three coronary arteries that supply blood to the heart. These coronary arteries are present on the surface of the heart and comprise of the left and right coronary arteries. The left coronary artery starts as a major vessel known as the left main coronary artery, which divides into the left anterior descending and the left circumflex arteries. The right coronary artery is a single vessel that supplies the back and lower portions of the heart. Most heart attacks are equally distributed between the left anterior descending and the right coronary arteries. Occlusion of the left circumflex is less common. Patients presenting with occlusions of the left anterior descending and the right coronary artery present quite differently. The occluded artery is easily distinguished on the EKG. A good doctor is not only able to diagnose a heart attack, but he will also be able to diagnose which part of the heart muscle is affected.

The left anterior descending is often the called the "widow maker," as it involves damage to a very large part of the heart muscle. "The Accountant" was having a heart attack involving the "widow maker."

Immediately upon seeing the large elevation of the ST-segments in the EKG, the paramedics knew that this was a big one.

"The Accountant," Victor, had no significant medical history except reflux esophagitis. But as the EKG demonstrated, this was not reflux disease. There was no doubt. Grace informed the paramedics that she had given Victor aspirin and nitroglycerin. In my conversations with Grace this morning, she said that the paramedics snapped at her for administering the nitroglycerin, stating that this would cause a drop in blood pressure.

The nitroglycerin aside, the paramedics clearly understood the fantastic role Grace had played. They were amazed at her diagnosis and the very clear thinking she had demonstrated in giving aspirin, checking the blood pressure and promptly calling 911. More lifesaving labor by Grace was to follow.

Grace was not allowed to travel in the ambulance as it sped out. She inquired where the ambulance was going. The paramedics informed her that it would be to Coral Community Hospital – her father practiced there for 40 years and was the Chief of Staff. She knew well that Coral Community Hospital was a very small hospital and would not be the right place for Victor who was having a massive heart attack.

Grace had known about angioplasty but had no idea how it could be life-saving for treating heart attacks. This was almost 10 years ago and there was not too much public awareness of Primary PCI. But she knew very lucidly that Coral Community Hospital was a very small hospital and she inferred that it was not the right place for Victor who was clearly facing a life-threatening emergency.

She confronted the paramedics head on and inquired why Victor was not being taken to Bayside Medical Center.

I do not know precisely what transpired. My inference is that the paramedics immediately recognized this to be the right decision and they promptly decided to proceed to Bayside Medical Center.

If Victor lives today, it is because of how brilliant Grace was and how clearly she thought and acted amidst this horrible emergency. I am not at all suggesting confrontations with EMS; in fact, nowadays none is needed, as almost always, the paramedics will proceed to the Primary PCI center. However, this is not a guarantee and I believe an educated patient and his loved ones can state this request to the paramedics. It is with little hesitation that I can state that a patient with a heart attack will have better outcomes at a Primary PCI hospital and that every effort should be made to take the patient there. At smaller hospitals, the most likely therapy would have been the use of a thrombolytic agent or the clot-buster. Or, the ER physician at Coral Community Hospital would have made efforts to transfer the patient to Bayside Medical Center. Clearly, there would be delays. You know why delays are detrimental to the patient with a heart attack. I am confident that you also know by now how there will always be a race against time when you or a loved one is having a heart attack. Keep in your mind, the absolute dictum that every minute counts, both for survival as well as to preserve the heart muscle.

You will learn in the book how thrombolysis is still used in several hospitals in the country and how we are rapidly moving away from its use. Thrombolytic drugs were a major revolution in Cardiology a few decades ago and they completely changed the management of heart attacks. They ushered in a revolution. Death rates were reduced and we had prompt agents that could quickly dissolve the clot and keep the vessel open. It modernized how heart attacks were treated everywhere in the world. Today, with Primary PCI and short D2B times, a similar transformation is occurring and we are benefiting from the lessons learned with use of thrombolytics.

Thrombolytic therapy was compared with Primary PCI in large clinical trials and the results were astounding. Primary PCI reduced death, strokes and recurrence of heart attack. It also reduced the chances of bleeding that are a major complication of thrombolytic therapy. Bleeding can even occur in the brain and be fatal. I was a medical resident in New York, in 1984, when thrombolytic therapy was just beginning. Our second patient was a VP of a major bank. He reached the ER with a massive heart attack and he made a fantastic recovery with the "magic" thrombolytic agent. Tragically, the same night, he died from a massive intracranial bleeding.

The switch from thrombolytic therapy to Primary PCI can be exemplified by learning from the British experience. Ten years ago, almost

90% of patients in the U.K. were treated by thrombolytic therapy. Today, almost 99% are treated with Primary PCI. These numbers are almost as impressive for our country where we had greater challenges of a massive country and five times the population.

Today, there are two situations where thrombolytic therapy is still used. 1) In cases where there is more than a 60-minute delay in reaching a hospital; 2) No PCI is available – this happens in developing countries. Another major drawback relates to the time window when thrombolytics are able to act. It is much shorter than for PCI. Therefore, poorer countries face a double dilemma – PCI is not available and the poor infrastructure delays presentation and makes thrombolytic therapy less effective.

How does all this relate to Grace and Victor? Events at the small Coral Community Hospital would have been totally different than at the PCI facility, Bayside Medical Center. Let us closely examine the events. I urge you to read carefully as you must understand this scenario and avoid getting trapped in it yourselves. At the small community hospital, there would first be the patient assessment, registration and insurance verification. Another EKG would be performed. Blood tests would be sent. A call would have to be made to the cardiologist on call. Often, it will be a while before the cardiologist calls back. How long do you think these events take? A good guess would be 60 minutes up to this point. Do these 60 minutes increase the chance of death? Is there a likelihood of permanent and life-long damage to your heart muscle from the delay in restoring the blood flow in the coronary artery? You know now that the answer to both questions is a resounding "Yes." With every precious minute that is lost, there is a greater likelihood of death and damage of the heart muscle.

I am sure the reality is now hitting you and that you understand the critical importance of not ending up with a heart attack, in a small hospital. A decade ago, it did not matter; the only option was thrombolytic therapy. The most effective treatment today is urgent Primary PCI. You must know this and end up in a Primary PCI hospital. This is what happened to Victor because Grace was smart.

This discussion also illustrates another life-saving matter. You must not self- transport during a heart attack. Never. Even a short drive must be resisted. The paramedics will diagnose and manage complications and take you to the Primary PCI hospital. This is your best chance of survival. It has been a legislative battle in various communities ensuring that the patient with a heart attack should go to the Primary PCI hospital. This advantage is lost if you have someone drive you to the nearest hospital. This is a complete fallacy. In 2019, what are the two best steps to save your life from a heart attack?

– CALL 911 AND TAKE ASPIRIN.

Just think how easy it was for Grace to fall into the trap of going to

Coral Community Hospital. It was just a few blocks away! Instead of calling 911, she could have opted to drive to this hospital.

There is no way to predict the outcome in the community hospital except that it would have been inferior to going directly to the Primary PCI hospital. Of course, it is entirely possible that the delay in reaching the Primary PCI hospital would have been catastrophic. Victor may have died!

We have lost about 60 minutes at the small hospital, most of this in silly matters such as registration and insurance verification. Further delays can be expected and they depend upon the decision to either transfer the patient or to administer thrombolytic therapy.

I must not make disparaging remarks about small, community hospitals. Many of these are excellent and they provide a fantastic service. But in 2019, they are not the place to be if you are having a heart attack. Let me provide you with more insights into the likely events had Victor ended up in Coral Community Hospital. The ER physician would have needed to make a tough decision – to either give thrombolytic therapy or to transfer to Bayside Medical Center. At the small, community hospital, both of these are correct options. And both are inferior to Primary PCI that would be performed if Victor reached (as he did) Bayside Medical Center. Today, the most likely option will be a transfer to Bayside Medical Center and I am certain that this would be a part of the protocol for treating heart attack patients at Coral Community Hospital. This situation occurs at most community hospitals in the country today – for patients with a heart attack, there would be an assigned pathway. This is your best chance and it involves delays. That could extinguish your life or make your life one of restrictions. You get it now – are you better prepared already for your heart attack? And to survive it?

We need to examine the two pathways at Coral Community hospital so that you can fully understand some of the decision points and the relevant issues.

In the first scenario, you receive thrombolytic therapy. Chances are you will get Tenecteplase, a superb, third generation, thrombolytic agent. It is known to have the highest rate of re-canalizing the blocked artery. This would occur in about 80% of cases. If it opens the artery, there will be immediate relief in the chest pain and the EKG will improve. In the 20% or so of situations where it does not open the artery, you need an urgent angioplasty. This makes the situation very complicated. The present-day strategy is to administer the thrombolytic agent and transfer to the Primary PCI hospital. We call this a pharmaco-invasive strategy. Invasive, as almost every patient that receives thrombolytic therapy requires a further cardiac catheterization procedure. It is similar in technique to an angioplasty, but it is the simple visualization of the coronary artery to search for blockages. In almost 80-90% of cases, further angioplasty is required after the thrombolytic therapy. You are shocked! As you should be. Why should one ever end up in a small hospital then? It is now obvious to you why thrombolytic therapy is inferior to Primary PCI and how you can avoid this thrombolytic option by simply calling 911 than by driving to a nearby, small hospital. I have tried not to further frighten you with details such as complications of bleeding with the thrombolytic agent. Or with further bad news that about 30% of the arteries that initially open up with the drug, end up re-occluding within the next 24 hours. This is why the patient who gets thrombolytic therapy must be transferred to a PCI hospital.

Imagine how awful the situation is in poorer countries! They have a heart attacks, they risk their lives by self-transporting themselves. Even at a major hospital, there are further delays in receiving treatment, which is often thrombolytic. This is all what they receive in the majority of poor country. You now understand my statement, "your outcome with a heart attack depends on your zip code". I also mentioned about our being fortunate in the United States. Our fate with a heart attack is so much better in the United States. It should be natural for you to immediately get scared about getting a heart attack when you are traveling out of the country. Or, while relaxing on a cruise? These are all relevant questions.

Let us examine the second pathway at the small, community hospital. The ER physician is smart, the PCI hospital is not too far (the requirement is for a driving time < 60 minutes), and he decides to transfer you for PCI. Hopefully, there will an ambulance immediately available. Sometimes, it is not. There are often delays as this is a lower priority than trauma or a heart attack in the field. For whatever reasons, there are almost always delays in transferring a heart attack patient from one hospital to the other – almost always, the response time is slower than for reaching a patient who is having a heart attack. All these delays will hurt you, both in the short and the long run. As efficiency has improved, patients who are being transferred for a PCI often bypass the ER. But there is enormous variability in this situation. This setting notwithstanding, you are in a sub-optimal pathway than heading straight to the Primary PCI facility.

Let us revisit some of these important issues to ensure your full comprehension. If you have a heart attack and you end up in a non-PCI hospital, you will either get thrombolytic therapy or be transferred to the Primary PCI hospital. Both options are clearly inferior to reaching the Primary PCI hospital in the first place. It is as simple as this. Imagine your concentration and attention to minute details as you are planning your retirement with a Financial Planner. If you screw up a little bit, it will cost you. Perhaps, you will end up taking Carnival Cruise Line for a cruise instead of Princess that you really wanted. Is this really a big deal? In the larger scheme of things, it is trivial. Let me teach you a big deal. You have a heart attack and you end up in a small hospital. This is a big deal. You could die. You could have serious complications such as a bleeding. Or none of these bad events happen; you are lucky and you survive. But there is damage to your heart muscle. You cannot play tennis forever or walk up two flights of stairs. This is a big deal.

You are already feeling glad you bought this book!

It is such a pity that these issues are not discussed in public forums and done so frequently. Why has it been left to me to reveal all these mysteries? Is this subject not as important as planning your retirement and your children's education? I hope that you are now beginning to appreciate the selection of the title of the book. I can assure you it will become even more poignant in the next few chapters. You must foresee the eventuality of a heart attack. Of the hundreds of patients that I have treated in almost 15 years, none thought they would have a heart attack. What makes you immune?

I want to pick up the true story of the remarkable Grace and how her genius saved her husband's life. The paramedics informed her that they were headed to Bayside Medical Center and that she could follow the ambulance, if she wanted.

Victor was already in a cubicle in the ER when Grace reached the hospital. He had already changed into the hospital gown and the nurse was telling him about the angioplasty. He needed to sign the Consent Form before she administered morphine for the chest pain. The paramedics had already told Victor that he would be having an urgent angioplasty. Grace and Victor discussed the options briefly and Victor promptly signed the consent. There was no doubt in their minds that this was the best option.

My beeper went off at 5:47 a.m., a minute or so after the ER physician had seen Victor's EKG. Bayside Medical Center is located very close to our home, so there was no great rush. Yet, I had made it a practice to reach the cath lab ahead of the on-call team. This triggered a greater sense of urgency in the team. The ER physician had described both the EKG and the patient very accurately. Victor looked very unwell but exactly as a patient with a massive heart attack involving the Left Anterior Descending Coronary Artery should look. This is a very large artery that supplies a major portion of the heart muscle that is now jeopardized. The on-call team had responded promptly and they had quickly prepared Victor for the procedure. I began quickly by first identifying all three coronary arteries. This first step, the coronary angiography precedes coronary angioplasty. It involves the visualization of the three coronary arteries with dye that shows the filling of these blood vessels. Two separate, pre-shaped catheters are used to cannulate the left and the right coronary arteries.

Victor's coronary angiography showed a normal left main (LMCA), a normal left circumflex (LCX), but a 100% occluded left anterior descending (LAD) coronary artery. The right coronary artery (RCA) was completely normal. It was a straightforward decision to open this blocked artery and to place a stent at the site of the occlusion. It needed to be done urgently.

As difficult as this may seem, this situation is far easier than the angioplasty that was needed to save Carlos's life. His circumstances were so much more challenging, and his entire procedure had been done on a heart that had stopped beating.

I advanced a tiny guide wire to cross the blocked LAD. After this, I used an extraction catheter to suction out the blood clot. This retrieved a big chunk of clot. This process immediately restored flow to the occluded vessel. Victor was immediately relieved. His chest pain was all gone. I then placed the coronary stent, a large, drug- coated one, at the site of the residual blockage. The vessel was as good as new.

This completely and immediately restored flow to Victor's occluded left anterior descending coronary artery. Medically, this represents cessation of the heart attack. As soon as blood rushes to the heart muscle, the cells receive oxygen and regain their normal function. Victor had absolute and complete relief of chest pain. His heart muscle was normal. The introducer sheaths in the right groin were removed in the cath lab after the procedure, and by 3 p.m., he was out of bed and walking.

As has been my practice for more than 25 years, I immediately went to speak to the patients' relatives after the procedure. This was when I first met Grace. She stated that she had seen me rushing into the cath lab about 20 minutes before and had presumed that I was the interventional cardiologist. I was intrigued and asked her how she knew that I was the doctor since I was rushing in scrubs without my white coat. She instantly replied that her father was a doctor, that she had seen many doctors, so she knew when she saw one! I told her that Victor was doing fine now after I had fixed the vessel and aborted the heart attack. But that he did sustain a big heart attack to begin with. I further informed her that I had placed a stent in the artery that had been occluded, and the heart muscle showed no visible sign of damage. Based upon the findings of the treated artery and the normal heart muscle, I told Grace that I expected Victor to do quite well.

I then asked her to tell me what had happened that morning.

In the cath lab, while doing the procedure, we mildly sedate the patient. Deeper sedation is often not required, as the cardiologist may require the patient to take a deep breath or to cough. In his mildly sedated state, Victor had mentioned about taking aspirin and nitroglycerin that his wife had given him. I was curious to know from Grace about what she had done and how she had reacted when Victor first complained.

Please read carefully as this paragraph may contribute to saving your life.

Grace mentioned that there was no doubt in her mind that Victor was having a heart attack. She did tell me about the reflux and the Gaviscon. I asked her then, as well as this morning, why she was so sure that this was a heart attack? Had she seen a heart attack before? How was she so certain? She mentioned that Victor was cold, pale, complaining of severe pressure in the middle of his chest, and that he was sweating profusely. Somewhat quizzically, she asked me, "What else could it be? It had to be a heart attack."

This was a stunning revelation from a patient's relative. How I wish more patients could react this way and demonstrate intellect and quick reaction in the middle of a catastrophe.

Compare Grace to Anna, Carlos's wife. She was fumbling and incoherent; she asked her brother to come to the ER, but forgot to tell him which hospital. Grace was, as you understand, truly amazing. So, what is the lesson here? It would be beyond the scope of this book to teach how one should stay calm in adversity. That is not what I am attempting here. But it is quite possible to observe more closely and to act immediately. Grace showed astute observation, clear thinking and prompt execution. In the forthcoming chapters, I will mention about how self-denial creates barriers in the prompt recognition of symptoms. That can happen more to the patient, perhaps, the loved one is less affected, although there is enormous variability about this observation.

The clear message of this case is that the patient and the family are very important contributors in saving a life from a heart attack. We are greatly advancing STEMI care after getting a 911 call, but we have a long way to go to make a patient understand the urgency to make the 911 call.

How Grace described Victor's condition is an absolutely classic presentation of a heart attack for the following reasons. Victor was 63. Here are two red flags. Heart attacks occur more in men who are in their middle age. An accountant would normally have a stressful job. Although this was September and beyond the frenzied tax-filing period, I have no doubt that Victor led a stressful life. The role of stress is important in causing heart attacks, and I will deal with this important subject later. A third and major factor why this may be a heart attack: Victor had been a heavy smoker.

In case of heart attacks, we relate to risk factors that cause a heart attack. This topic is exhaustively discussed in numerous sections of the book. There are numerous predisposing factors that cause a heart attack. You have already encountered three. Simply put, there were three good reasons that Victor was having a heart attack. Three reasons to explain, "What else could it be." Call it intellect, previous readings or a wife's intuition. Grace honed on to this most accurately.

Smoking is a very big risk factor. The remaining three major risk factors include high blood pressure, diabetes, and high levels of fats, "lipids," in the blood. The role of risk factors is paramount in causing heart attacks. Beyond these major risk factors are a few (relatively) minor risk factors. These include the male sex, a family history of coronary artery disease, and stress. Every few months, there are scientific reports of newer contributing risk factors, such as pollution.

However, let us focus on the clearly proven risk factors. When you now begin to look at it in this methodical fashion, Victor was a sitting duck for a heart attack!

Is this your profile? Are you a sitting duck too?

You must identify the Victor in your own life, whether it is you, the male reader, or it is the other male members that display this pattern. Sit back right now for a moment and do a quick analysis. Who fits this pattern among your immediate male relatives - your brother, your father, or your grandfather? This is a prudent way for you to begin. Let us first focus on the more vulnerable one, the male sex. I will be presenting female patients subsequently and in great detail.

To illustrate the most susceptible patient and to help you quickly identify if you could be at risk, I carefully selected two male patients first.

Carlos and Victor, the two male patients who were having a heart attack should help you identify whether you or your loved one is a potential casualty.

Between these risk factors, it is my belief that diabetes possibly represents the most malignant risk factor because it is a lifelong disease despite management. Diabetes is also a multi-organ disease that increases fat deposition in various arteries including in the coronary vessels. The metabolic changes that occur from glucose and sugar imbalance in diabetic patients also affect nerve endings. Because of this, these nerves are somewhat numbed for pain. As a result, diabetics will often not experience the same level of chest pain while having a heart attack. We also know that there are two types of diabetic patients, those that require insulin, and those that are managed by diet and non-insulin therapies. The insulin-dependent diabetics are the more severe patients that often develop coronary artery disease in their later stages of life. In my evaluation of patients with chest pain, after I have understood the description of the chest pain, I proceed to inquire about the presence of risk factors. Amongst these, I first ask about diabetes because of the supreme understanding that it is the most menacing risk factor for coronary artery disease.

A difficulty arises since several patients first find out that they are diabetics in the middle of a crisis, such as a heart attack. It is not uncommon to find a patient with a heart attack who had never known he was diabetic and is found to have diabetes during the hospitalization for the heart attack.

Irrespective, I emphatically search for the presence of diabetes in any patient who presents with chest pain.

The next big risk factor is smoking. Of course, most patients will underreport this habit; many will state that they are smokers but had given up the habit. Usually, they sheepishly admit that they gave it up last week! Smoking, because of its continual administration of nicotine, is one of the most potent causes of coronary artery disease. Unlike diabetes, it can be entirely eliminated. Smokers who give up smoking for a year can eliminate smoking as a risk factor entirely. One of the tragedies of modern management of coronary artery disease is that we have made it extremely easy for patients to return to their negligent lifestyles. Two decades ago, a heart attack required two weeks of hospitalization. This longer hospitalization provided a deeper opportunity to interact with the patient and the family and it enabled recommendations for lifestyle changes and for risk factor modification, during the critical time period when the patient was more pliable to reflecting and trying to make these changes. My patients with heart attack go home on day 3, and several on day 2. It is simply too easy for them once they have survived. Their psyche and intellect have not been rudely awakened, and the price of a heart attack appears too little to pay for giving up their smoking indulgence.

One of my saddest memories as an interventional cardiologist was a patient, I took care of two decades ago. I remember him vividly after so long. Those days, my life was one of a busy interventional cardiologist who performed numerous complex angioplasty procedures each day. That morning, I had taken care of a middle-aged gentleman whose procedure was extremely difficult. He had bilateral amputations. I did a very difficult procedure from the arm, during which I had to navigate with multiple catheters the very tortuous coronary arteries. The patient had previously had a bypass surgery, and I ended
up having to place stents in a previously bypassed graft. Later that evening, as I walked to the parking lot of the hospital, I saw the same patient in a wheel chair, and smoking.

Our country has made strides in reducing the rates of smoking that has also decreased heart disease. However, we can do more. The rates of smoking in teenagers and women are simply too high.

I would like to share a personal observation that I believe made me a much better doctor. Between 1999 and 2000, when I was the President of the American Heart Association in South Florida, I did much public speaking about Heart Disease. For the Board of the American Heart Association that met each month, I created the Mehta Medical Minute that discussed issues related to preventing heart disease. This was a very different discipline than performing angioplasty. But this tenure as a cardiologist discussing prevention clearly elevated my intellect and it enormously contributed to my developing a more mature and balanced perspective about heart disease. I sincerely share these "mature" thoughts with you in a humble effort to help you.

Smoking cessation is of paramount importance after angioplasty. In particular, after angioplasty that was done to treat a heart attack. The role of counseling, nicotine substitutes, and other forms of therapy is crucial. Smoking cessation is an absolute requirement. Sometimes, I wish that there were more insurance penalties for smokers. Of course, this is difficult to implement, and I also remind myself to stay away from political minefields in my writing endeavors. Irrespective, patients with a heart attack who continue to smoke – for them, it is only a matter of when the disease will recur, not how!

Grace recollects a blood test of Victor's that showed borderline blood lipids, but he did not have high blood pressure. So here we have a middle-aged male with a long-standing history of smoking. Chest pain in this situation is highly suggestive of a heart attack.

So then, reverting to Grace, "what else could it be?"

The description of mid sternal chest pain with accompanying difficulty of breathing, sweating, and being pale are absolute classic presentations.

There is one more worrying feature that was present in Victor's heart attack. His symptoms occurred in the early morning hours. This is another common occurrence. A large number of heart attacks occur in the early morning hours for a variety of reasons. The underlying mechanism of a heart attack is a total or almost total blockage of one or more coronary arteries by the presence of blood clots. Often, these blood clots deposit at the site of previous fatty deposits inside the coronary artery. These fatty "plaques" result from the effects of unmitigated risk factors over many years.

A fatty plaque, that has been stable, despite enlarging in size, has a layer of protective tissue that covers it. Because of some precipitating factors, this lining ruptures. This can happen during unusual physical activity, mental anguish and stress, cold weather, smoking, and from a host of other, as yet poorly understood, reasons. Once this protective barrier is broken, a patient that was previously stable, suddenly develops severe symptoms. This broken lining attracts the deposition of the blood cells that are known as platelets.

Let us take a moment to understand the platelets as they greatly contribute to the development of a heart attack. The platelets have both a protective effect and the destructive effect that causes heart attacks. It is the platelets that are responsible for a shielding clot development that heals wounds. In the case of a heart attack, however, the blood clot occludes a previously narrowed coronary artery.

The simple reason why angioplasty works more effectively than the clot busters is because it treats both the blood clot and the fatty plaque. In contrast, clot buster drugs only impact the blood clot and they have no effect on fatty deposits. It is this essential difference that has propelled the scientific recommendations of angioplasty being the preferred treatment for heart attacks.

The platelets are stickier in the early morning hours, and a broken protective layer provides an exposed surface for the active platelets to deposit and rapidly form a blood clot inside the lumen of the coronary artery. Besides, the activity of the platelets, other aspects of human physiology also contribute to more heart attacks in the early morning hours. When patients wake up, they have increased blood pressure and heart rate – these increase the chance of a heart attack. Facing the challenges on Monday mornings is also a classic for reasons of mental stress. The classic tale of a person having a heart attack while shoveling snow in the morning is because of the combined and deleterious effects of physical and mental stress and the cold weather.

One of the most potent blockers of platelet activation is the simple drug aspirin. This is a true lifesaver. The history of aspirin is fascinating. Its use dates back to Hippocrates and the Egyptians. In the modern age, Bayer was a pioneer in developing and promoting this drug. A young chemist, working for Bayer, Dr. Felix Hoffman, is recognized as the inventor of this wonder drug that treats fever and pain, and heart attacks! The latter benefit occurs as aspirin is a potent blocker of the platelets that form blood clots and result in heart attacks. The early use of aspirin in heart attacks is strongly endorsed for this precise reason.

The story of Rosie O'Donnell and her survival from a heart attack has created huge awareness about heart attacks and about the preventative effects of aspirin. Rosie O'Donnell was not at all aware of what was happening. She only had pain in her biceps for which she took aspirin. The next day, she saw a cardiologist and learned that one of her arteries was 99% blocked, and that she had sustained a heart attack.

In recounting the story of Victor, "the Accountant," it was truly not me, but Grace, who saved his life. She did this in three obvious ways. Firstly, through her intellect and education, she diagnosed the problem accurately. Secondly, she administered aspirin, the lifesaver.

The third reason requires more contemplation. During several moments of Victor's discomfort with the heart attack, he tended to moderate his symptoms. This is a very common occurrence.

Some of the brightest individuals can suddenly become naysayers and convince themselves, "heart attack won't happen to me."

Many patients also succumb to the temptation and they proceed with their planned activity instead of seeking help immediately.

Where is the doubt that Victor would rather be watching the Marlins play the Reds than be in a hospital bed?

Grace put an end to Victor's plans for the day. Both have since made three enjoyable trips to Cincinnati to enjoy the ball game with their friends.

Patients have amazing ways to show appreciation for their doctors. A few months after Victor's angioplasty, he invited my wife and I to the Gulfstream Park to enjoy horse racing. This was not an activity I would indulge in, but Grace promised, "I would enjoy the experience." As we entered the Park, we were stunned at the sight of hundreds of raucous fans screaming, "Go, Dr. Mehta, Go!"

Running in lane 8, was a fine colt, owned by Victor and Grace, who had been named, "Dr. Mehta" by Victor, in honor of the doctor that saved his life from a heart attack.

CHAPTER 3. THE BIRTHDAY GIFT OF LIFE

If you haven't got any charity in your heart, you have the worst kind of heart trouble.
Bob Hope

Both our children were in town. The Mehta family was going to have a wonderful birthday dinner celebration for my wife, Shoba. It was September 13. We chose the delightful Café Abbracci in Coral Gables and looked forward to an evening of relaxation. But there was a snag. I had not been able to change my STEMI on-call. But then, this had become a norm, and this was one of the many ways that I was balancing the personal and STEMI life. This groundwork included placing a duffel bag in all three cars, each containing a pair of scrubs, sneakers, and socks. Another remarkable, military-style, exercise that I instituted was to always place my scrub shoes, socks, and the car keys under the easy chair in the living room. Till this day, 15 years later, when on call, the shoes and keys   can always be found there. The wallet, hospital ID, the laminated hospital parking permit, and the white coat were always on the backseat. Since I slept in scrubs, changing clothes was no issue. Just like that day, whenever we went out to dinner or to meet friends, we always went in separate cars, just in case I had to rush out for a STEMI.

This is exactly what happened on this day, and another family celebration was ruined. Worst of all, the STEMI call came at precisely the moment when Shoba was opening her birthday gift that I had bought her.

A most remarkable part was that neither my wife nor our children registered any protest whatsoever. I have always deeply appreciated this family support. It has been the main sustenance in the furious professional life that I have maintained over 15 years. After the children went away to college, my wife, who is a homemaker, would often drive with me as I went to one of the four hospitals where I took STEMI calls. The calls were one week at a time, alternating between different hospitals. I selected these hospitals based on numerous criteria that I will describe subsequently. Although Shoba stated that she was providing company to me, I suspect the main reason was for her to ensure that I drove safely!

I have openly acknowledged that driving fast to do a STEMI at 3 AM is far more challenging than the procedure itself.

My driving record during the first five years of STEMI on call was abysmal, punctuated by speeding violations and accidents – I could devote an entire book reviewing these misadventures.

For 15 years, Shoba has said the same two short sentences to me each time as I rushed to take care of a patient with a heart attack, "Drive safely. Say your prayers."

To my family, I owe my lifelong appreciation for adjusting to the repeat and frequent violation of our sanity and the family order. Just about every family activity, be it social engagements, children's graduations, holiday events, and of course, their birthdays, got disrupted by a STEMI call.

As was this one.

I sped in my car and reached Bayside Medical Center in about 8 minutes – we never dined more than 10 minutes away from the hospital where I took call!

I had also learned an amazing discipline during these years. A STEMI procedure was like a blind date; there was no way for me to predict what or who I would confront. Often, it was a simple procedure that I gladly accepted with humility. Other times, I could have a 400 lb. patient where accessing the arteries became monumentally challenging. Particularly, while chasing a mandatory Door-to-Balloon time (D2B). There were a multitude of other challenges, such as delays by other members of the team, equipment failure, ER delays, and hundreds of technical variables that complicate the procedure.

In 15 years, no two procedures have been alike.

The habit that I practiced to prepare for the "blind date" was to immediately get into the car and begin driving to the hospital. This was the only event that I could control during a STEMI intervention. I had absolutely no control over traffic or the challenges that I mentioned above. This single discipline of jumping into the car as soon as I could has contributed much to my sanity and it has provided the stamina to maintain practice of a punishing profession. It also slowed (sadly, not eliminated) the traffic citations and accidents in recent years.

I was in for a rough ride on this auspicious day. Just about every trick of my trade needed to be executed, speedily and accurately.

Mr. Pedro Hernandez, then 75 years old, had presented to the emergency room with a massive heart attack and a cardiac arrest. His presentation was almost as dramatic as that of Carlos, with the real difference being that Pedro Hernandez was 75, as opposed to the younger Carlos.

I am sure the Hernandez family was expecting the worst and they would have accepted the loss of their loved one.

With Carlos, who was 48, the situation was totally different.

The similarity of both patients having a cardiac arrest ended at just that – the proceedings were dramatically different. Pedro was wide awake despite sedation and pain medication during the entire tormenting 30

32

minutes during which we needed to shock Pedro 18 times!

Repeatedly, despite the use of powerful drugs that can restore a normal rhythm, his heart pattern kept converting to the very dangerous and life-threatening ventricular fibrillation (VF). The treatment for this is delivering an electric shock to the heart with the defibrillator. This was also the malignant rhythm that we saw with Carlos. VF is the most common cause of death for patients with heart attack. The purpose of placing automated external defibrillator (AED) in public places is for use in such situations.

The surreal feature with Pedro was that he became alert immediately with each shock! He would attempt to sit up in a daze and we would restrain him. He was sedated but the powerful shocks broke through sedation. In between the shocks, he was incredibly lucid. This was most unusual but it helped me complete an audacious procedure.

From the ER, I accompanied him during the short transport to the cath lab. Just like Carlos, even during this brief transit, he was shocked thrice. The procedure became trickier for numerous reasons. One of the nurses was continually positioned with the defibrillator paddles in her hands ready to thump the patient's chest. Each time the shock was delivered, the patient was thrust upward, knocking the equipment off the table. We could not place patient constraints as that could injure his wrists during the violent lunges of the patient when shocked. Everyone had to step away from the table each time the shock was delivered. Therefore, each time the shock was delivered, the catheters and syringes became disassembled. Of course, I sutured the access sheaths, but the other catheters could not be firmly secured.

The patient had been treated with anti-arrhythmic drugs to break this rhythm. We had also corrected the electrolyte imbalances. But the VF was arising from another source - a critical lesion of the left main trunk of the coronary artery.

With the knowledge of the coronary anatomy from the previous chapter, you may have surmised how critical the occlusion of the left main can be – since the left main gives rise to the left anterior descending and the left circumflex, once the left main is blocked, there is no blood going to either of the branches. Two of the three branches are occluded and this is a catastrophic cardiac emergency. With a total occlusion of the left main, it was a surprise that Pedro was still alive. He was living off the circulation from his right coronary artery that was barely enough and this was resulting in recurrent V. Fib.

The treatment for left main disease is surgery to bypass both occluded branches. More recently, angioplasty for the left main is being performed at expert centers and it is mainly to treat patients that are unable to have surgery. Even then, this procedure is fraught with the possibility of sudden cardiac death and there are several other complications.

However, this procedure was done in 2005, when stenting of the left main was rare. I instinctively knew that the correct treatment was surgery. But in this precarious, life-threatening situation, surgery was simply not an option. It was a miracle that Pedro was still alive.

With each shock, the patient's death appeared imminent. A salvage angioplasty remained the only option. I took it.

I utilized a special catheter to cannulate the left coronary artery, remaining cautiously mindful of not causing further catheter-related injury and anticipating further VF. This needed to be done very quickly, which I did. But even in the few minutes it took me to stent this major vessel, the patient needed to be resuscitated twice!

Broadly, the angioplasty procedure was similar to the one for Carlos and as precarious. But the techniques were somewhat different. I was able to navigate the wire through the occluded left main and I performed an ultra-short balloon inflation to create some flow and to help me position the stent. This quick balloon inflation reestablished mild flow into the left coronary artery. But it also ended the vicious cycle of VF. I was now able to visualize the left main and I quickly deployed a large stent in the diseased segment of the left main coronary artery.

The miracle was done. It has been almost 11 years since that day, and Pedro has had no recurrence of the malignant rhythm that threatened his life. The patient made a phenomenal recovery. By the next morning, he was in the company of his grandchildren and walking with ease.

Over the last decade, an excellent clinical cardiologist, Dr. Shaykhar, has performed regular stress tests to look for any signs of recurrence. A few years ago, Mr. Hernandez had mild chest discomfort. I quickly performed a coronary angiography to evaluate the previously placed stent in the left main coronary artery. There was new disease in the   left anterior descending artery that was easily treated with an additional stent. The left main was widely patent.

Religiously, every 13th day of September, the patient's son calls me to express his father's gratitude and that of the large number of his children, grandchildren, and great grandchildren.

Through the marvelous procedure of primary PCI, Mr. Hernandez received a Birthday gift of life!

CHAPTER 4. THE BMW IS GONE!

Life is really simple, but we insist on making it complicated.
Confucius

October 30, 2010 was a remarkable day… for all the wrong reasons.

Throughout the afternoon and the evening, "super-cell" thunderstorm activity produced torrential rains and flash flooding in Miami. I was on call at Gateway Hospital, 15.3 miles from our home in Coconut Grove, Miami. The right decision should have been for me to drive to the hospital during one of the rain interruptions and sleep in at the hospital. But I was tired from a previous procedure and the on-call room was unappealing. So, I stayed at home, hoping that there would be no more emergencies.

Unfortunately, this was not the only wrong decision I made on that fateful day.

At 11:02 PM, when the hospital operator announced a STEMI, I was extremely concerned. The storm was at its worst, and I knew that several streets would be flooded. The correct decision should have been for me to drive my Volkswagen Touareg. With its higher engine platform, this would have been the safer option. My hospital ID, parking permits, and white coat were already in it. For whatever reason, I decided to switch cars. I have tormented over this terrible decision for years now and I wonder what contributed to this lack of judgment. I believe that I was more concerned about the brakes in the old Touareg. I felt that my son, Kabir's, (the book has been dedicated to him for his motivating influence) brand new BMW would be the safer option because of the brakes.

Of course, my wonderful wife accompanied me. We drove out cautiously, with me at the wheels.

The patient was a 42-year-old male with a massive anterior wall myocardial infarction.

Fortunately, there was minimal traffic. However, almost all roads, including I-95 were flooded. I drove extremely carefully, navigating cautiously through the puddles. Just before entering the I-95 ramp, the engine hesitated. This was strange, and worrisome. It was a brand-new car. Why the decelerating? I tried not to panic but I was alarmed. But I was about to reach the broad expressway, where the road would be in a better condition. I was also distracted and intensely focused on the young patient with the heart attack.

What I had not known was that the BMW has a completely electric transmission. It also has a very low engine platform and that any water escaping into the engine would completely disable the electric circuit.

On the highway, the car functioned perfectly, and I soon dismissed the sputter from my head. Fastidiously, I drove gently in the middle lane, which to me represented the safest of the three lanes. The windshield wipers were thrashing furiously. But I was making steady progress. I even called the hospital to get a status update on the patient who was en route from the ER. I was now midway and quite composed. With all my experience, I was fairly confident that I would overcome the "process" challenges and perform another life-saving "procedure" with relative calm.

This was a terrible miscalculation and a personal misfortune.

A small road, off the highway, leads to the hospital. Gateway Hospital has two buildings; both are located on elevated ramps that gently slope down to the road. Since the incident that I describe below, I have walked up the ramp and paused to inspect the area. It is strange that the flaw in this construction was never picked up. In a storm, the two ramps serve as a drain for water that gushes down from both and floods the small road.

On this fateful day, this precise phenomenon had occurred. The rush of water from both ramps had completely flooded this road, and I drove right into it. About midway into this flooded street, the car stalled and seized. I looked behind and judged that my chance of getting through the water were better by advancing than reversing.

To this day, I have no idea how I came to this conclusion. Either way, the end result may have been the same. I cranked the ignition and the car restarted. But now it was dragging. It barely moved another few yards before aborting. It was completely dead. The key would not even turn. All dash lights were dark. I tried a few times, but the engine would not start.

Even worse, the car was now stuck right at the junction where both ramps were pouring floodwater into the street.

Panic now set in, as I could not open the car door. There was enormous force of torrential water against both doors. I wondered what to do now. The water has rising and was already at the level of the window. I leaned towards the passenger seat and with both feet, pushed hard the driver side door with all the strength I could muster. Already, we had grabbed the essential contents from the car - my wallet, hospital ID, white coat and Shoba's handbag. The door yielded with this mighty push and water surged into the car. I stepped out of the car and dragged Shoba along. Out of the car, we somehow managed to get off the flooding street. From there, we ran to the side of the main building and climbed the stairs that lead into the hospital lobby.

Once inside the hospital, we both gathered our composure; Shoba went to the restroom, and I ran to the cath lab. As I ran past the security guard, I yelled at him to look out for the car we had left behind. I quickly changed into new scrubs and dabbed my hair dry. In the quiet moment as I scrubbed, I reminded myself to put the car mishap out of my mind and concentrate on the job at hand – a life had to be saved.

The angioplasty was routine and simple, and it took less than 10 minutes to stent the occluded artery and restore good flow to the vessel. The heart attack was aborted, and the patient was fully relieved of his chest pain.

The security guard had rushed back to the cath lab and told me, "Doc, I don't see any car!"

I was perplexed. Then, it struck me that in the rush, I must have miscommunicated to the guard about the location of the car. I rushed to the lobby where Shoba was waiting. The rain had paused, and we hurried out to look for the car. From the hospital porch, the flooded street could be well visualized.

The BMW was gone! It had submerged completely.

It took almost two hours before the tow truck finally came – it had been hectic for the towing company as they were responding to numerous accidents. It was a challenge   to guide the tow truck driver to where I thought our submerged BMW would have been. We tried for a long time, the heavy rains had resumed and the driver told us that he needed a bigger truck and that they needed for the rain to stop and for the water to recede.

I never saw the car again. It was totaled. We managed to recover most of its value through our insurance policy. The worst part of the story was confronting Kabir with the news. He responded magnanimously and expressed gratitude/relief at our safety. On his Christmas break, there was a new car waiting in the garage for him and I was unburdened of the guilt of losing the other one.

A few months later, I read, with great dismay, about flash floods in Beijing, China. I was appalled to read further details. Numerous cars had submerged outside the Beijing Railway station and 28 Chinese perished. There was a graphic description about the death of a young man who was trapped in his BMW. In his last moments, he kept calling his wife on his cell phone. With so many submerged vehicles, his car could not be spotted in the flooded street.

CHAPTER 5. HUMILITY

Humility is not thinking less of yourself; it's thinking of yourself less.
C.S. Lewis

Women seem to regularly save the lives of their husbands from heart attacks!

George Mandel, a very successful Miami attorney, may not have been alive were it not for his wife, Briana, and for her alertness and unruffled, presence of mind.

As he gently navigated his sailboat into the Key Biscayne marina, he experienced sudden, crushing chest pain and collapsed on the boat floor. Briana grabbed the wheel and hurriedly steered the boat into the dock. George was groggy but conscious. She inquired how he was doing as she swiftly anchored the ropes and secured the boat. Then, she turned her attention back to George. He was pale, sweaty, and gasping for air. Briana called 9-1-1 on her mobile phone.

She too, like Grace, the accountant's wife, accurately diagnosed a heart attack   and that is exactly what she told the 911 dispatcher who answered her call. The Key Biscayne EMS responded swiftly, and very shortly, they were at the site and on the boat. George was laid down on the boat, and the paramedics rapidly performed an EKG. They diagnosed the heart attack and immediately called the ER at Bayside Medical Center. The ER physician was provided a quick clinical update, including the vital signs. The paramedics provided a 7-minute ETA to the ER. In the ambulance, oxygen was administered, aspirin was given, and an intravenous placed. The quick ambulance ride was unremarkable, as was the short ER stop.

Over the last decade, considerable progress has been made in shortening D2B times while treating heart attacks. Each valuable minute saved in this process can contribute to both saving the patient's life and recovering his heart muscle.

Several early initiatives to reduce D2B times were the low-hanging fruit, and most hospitals in the United States were easily able to incorporate these essential changes. Further progress, not unexpectedly, has been more difficult, and this has required considerable collaboration between paramedics, ER, and the cath lab.

I compare a STEMI process to a 100 m X 4 relay race, in which 4 STEMI sprinters must act in perfect unison. These 4 STEMI partners include the patient, the paramedic, the ER physician, and the interventional cardiologist. As in a relay, where the baton must be precisely handed to the next runner, the care of the STEMI patient must be seamlessly passed on to the next member. A slow response by any member affects the D2B time, and this can hugely affect a patient's outcome.

One of the challenges of treating a heart attack patient is the sudden and unpredictability of events. A patient who may appear completely stable has VF or heart block that can cause death. To avoid any such or other complication, the D2B time must be reduced as much as possible.

Over the years, several friends and patients have questioned me about my mad pursuits during a STEMI intervention.

I provide a simple answer, rather I pose a straightforward question – if this were your father, how quickly would you want me to open his artery?

Should it be in the mandated 90 minutes or should it be sooner? This changes everything, and the answer has often come back as 80, 70, 60, 50 minutes. Or, often the answer is "in as short a time as possible." See, how easy it is to understand my life?

Although I have not missed a D2B mandate in several years, the profound desire to reduce D2B time has always kept me on a treadmill, the speed of which is controlled by my conscience.

A large, presently unsolved puzzle pertains to whether a patient with a heart attack being brought in by an ambulance should even stop in the emergency room. We refer to this as ER bypass. The proponents of this process, including myself, firmly believe that an overwhelming majority of the patients can bypass the emergency room and thereby save valuable minutes. This must be achieved with a caveat, that of the cath lab team and the interventional cardiologist being ready to accept the patient. In some hospitals in Puerto Rico, where I helped create a nation-wide heart attack program, we found an ingenious solution. There is a large green light in the emergency room; they press a button to lights the green sign. This enables clear communication and a signal to bypass the ER. Proponents of ER bypass point to the enormous benefits of saving precious D2B minutes. They also point out the major events that occur in the ER that has nothing to do with patient care, which includes patient registration and insurance verification. We simply must be intelligent to avoid such delays, and I am sure more efficient solutions can be found to perform these ancillary functions. Of course, a crashing patient is a different matter, and yes, the patient would need urgent treatment in the ER. In fact, to stabilize such patients   is far more important than chasing a D2B time. However, an overwhelming majority of patients are stable and should proceed directly to the cath lab. I believe that the practice pioneered at the Minnesota Heart Institute by Dr. Timothy Henry and his team is the most appropriate. In this method, the patient is quickly evaluated without being taken off the ambulance stretcher. This simple, yet extremely well devised strategy saves precious minutes. If you have ever watched a patient being placed into a monitored hospital bed, you will clearly understand this to be a time-consuming activity. To transfer a patient, from an ambulance stretcher onto the bed, and sometimes, off again, should be avoided, whenever possible. Of course, several ER beds can be used to transport the patients, yet the entire exercise seems redundant, in particular for stable patients with a heart attack where speed is critical in opening the artery. Finally, nobody in the world knows better how to take care of a heart attack patient than the team in the cath lab.

My team and I were ready in the cath lab to treat George. As he was being prepped, I quickly assessed him, examined to his heart and lungs, and spoke briefly to Briana to reassure her. Thirty minutes later, after performing a smooth STEMI intervention, I was back with her for a more relaxed conversation.

Almost 8 years have passed, and George continues to thrive. On last year's New Year's Eve, he invited my family and me to a celebration party at the Ritz Carlton Hotel in Key Biscayne. Unknown to me, some honor had been planned. Of course, I was on call- why else would this description be in this book!

At almost the precise moment when my wife and our son Kabir were going to drive (in separate cars) to the party, the hospital beeped me for a STEMI. Within a minute, with practiced ease, the Mehta family discussed various options.

Sadly, the family determined on the worst one!

Shoba and Kabir did not want to attend the party without me. Instead, they succumbed to Dr. Mehta's gallant remark, "It will take me 15 minutes to do the procedure, and then we'll go in and ring in the New Year."

Promptly, the Mehtas jumped into Kabir's new car; however, I sank into deep gloom as I called the cath lab. The patient was in profound shock, and he had sustained a cardiac arrest. He had also been intubated and he was on multiple medications to maintain his heart function. This was not good news. I simply did not have the courage to relay this information to my family. Anyway, since we were already more than midway to the hospital, it was too late to reverse course. Besides, who knew, this could be my lucky day, and the miraculous procedure of angioplasty would quickly save this patient's life.

Probably the last remaining big challenge, in the management of heart attacks, is the care of a patient who presents with shock. We call this cardiogenic shock. Almost every top cardiology research center is working on improving outcomes of patients with heart attack and accompanying shock. We refer to shock as an inability to maintain the pumping function of the heart. This leads to insufficient supply of oxygen to vital body organs. The blood pressure is simply not enough to enable blood flow to these organs as a result of the failing heart muscle.

The first line of management for this failing heart is to intravenously administer drugs to whip the failing heart. These drugs are known as inotropes. Beyond these drugs are innovative methods to beef up the heart muscle, the myocardium.

Innovative heart support devices are used for this purpose. Two of the more commonly used devices to support the failing heart include the intra-aortic balloon pump, and the Impella, Left Ventricular Assist Device (LVAD). Both are highly invasive procedures and have relative merits and demerits. Although the intra-aortic balloon pump (IABP) has been used for several decades, and deployment has become considerably easier, some recent research questions its effectiveness. The Impella catheter, by comparison, has been found to be more effective.

Death rates from shock that complicates a heart attack can be extremely high, and as much as 60-80%. Cardiogenic shock, unresponsive to inotropes, is a harbinger of grave prognosis.

Both these life-saving devices must be inserted through the groin using either the right or left femoral artery. Heart attack angioplasty can be performed by either accessing the right or the left groin or via the right or left wrist. Several important changes in the access route have occurred in the last few years. In the unfortunate event of your ever needing this procedure, this may be one of the first questions posed to you by the cardiologist. Let me educate you about this important topic.

The major advantage of performing the procedure from the groin is the ability to approach the large femoral artery. Accessing a large artery has several benefits. A large artery allows easy placement of devices and navigation of catheters. Using left ventricular support devices, such as IABP and Impella, is only possible through the femoral route.

The navigation route is as follows – the right and left femoral arteries lead into the aorta, the biggest artery in our body. The aorta ascends across the abdomen and the thorax and ends up in the pumping chamber of the heart, the left ventricle. The two coronary arteries arise before the aorta ends in the left ventricle.

An alternate approach is to access the coronary arteries from the radial arteries in the wrist. More recently, the ulnar artery on the side of the little finger is also being used as an access site, but this is less common. There are two advantages of using the radial artery – it reduces bleeding and the patient is able to ambulate earlier. Because of these important reasons, patients seem to prefer the use of the wrist rather than the groin.

The easy answer, if ever confronted with this option, should be allowing this to be the operator's decision. Many interventional cardiologists are better trained with the femoral route, and they believe that accessing a larger artery is more advantageous. On the other hand, wrist access is becoming more prevalent, and your operator may desire this option. Since a STEMI intervention needs to be performed speedily, a physician's comfort with the technique is paramount. Therefore, the recommendation is to let this be the operator's choice.

Beyond learning about the groin or right access site, what is some additional information that you should know?

Several hospitals that perform primary PCI will readily provide information about their STEMI performance. There are a few relevant metrics to gauge them. As a first one, it is the availability to perform 24/7 STEMI interventions. Most institutions will reply in the affirmative to this query.

Additional questions may be asked to the institution: their D2B times, the success rate and their relative ranking of the hospital's STEMI program in the community. As an example, Gateway Hospital ranks high with an average D2B time of 63 minutes.

I must caution you right away – the information about the D2B time may be an over- simplification, as a D2B time may not necessarily mean the best outcome!

There are some healthy questions being raised about the validity of D2B times in the overall care of a patient with heart attack. Several physicians correctly point to the myopic focus on D2B times. They refer to the true ischemic time as a better parameter. This may indeed be correct. Allow me to explain.

A true ischemic time would be the overall time during which the heart muscle is under assault. It is calculated from when the chest pain begins and not from when the patient walks through the door of the hospital. Does this not make more sense?

It also places a critical onus on the patient and his or her ability to recognize and respond to chest pain. After all, if the patient has had chest pain for 6 hours before calling 9-1-1, there is not much use for me to drive at 90 mph to save the patient's life! The chances are that after six hours of chest pain, there has already been severe damage of the heart muscle.

At this juncture, I want to provide you a clear game plan about foreseeing your Primary PCI and that of your loved one.

At its starting point, you must investigate, and know for certain, which is the nearest hospital to you that performs primary PCI. You could even plot it out on the map and speculate the driving distance and the driving times.

Beyond securing the aspirin and statin (drugs used for lowering blood cholesterol), this is my second-best recommendation that may save your life.

Not only should you know this hospital, it may be a good idea for you to visit it and ask pertinent questions that you have now understood?

You may actually want to do it for your elderly family members.

Each may benefit from this information.

Like your physician's phone number, this information should be visibly stored.

Although there is every possibility that you would be taken to the right hospital, to get more information about this institution is of real benefit to you.

Gradually, as we proceed further in the book, I will compile for you a complete Check List that will help you to "plan for your heart attack… and survive it." As a start, know about your Primary PCI hospital. Be sure it is a solid operation and not a mere marketing ploy by the hospital. Make this exercise as deliberate as your hunt for the right school in your tax district.

My worst fears, with the patient that I was treating on New Year's Eve, were coming true. I quickly deposited my family into the meager physician lounge and rushed to the cath lab. It did not take any great effort to recognize that the patient was beyond grave. The blood pressure was barely palpable despite maximal therapy with drugs, the inotropes. The patient had heart and lung failure and the artificial breathing machine had been inserted. There was bleeding at the entry site where the breathing tube was entering into the mouth. The patient was completely unconscious and his pupils were sluggish – this is a very poor sign for survival.

I had an enormous challenge ahead of me. I confronted every possible obstacle and every component of the angioplasty procedure, was extremely difficult. As a start, pulses in both femoral arteries were completely absent. I needed access to both femoral arteries, one to do angioplasty and the other for inserting an intra-aortic balloon pump (IABP) to support the blood pressure. This required numerous arterial sticks with the insertion needle. Since the artery could not be felt, the needle sticks were missing the artery. The knowledge of anatomy had to be relied upon – however, the patient was markedly obese and the normal anatomical landmarks were lost. There was also severe disease that involved all the arteries that I need to traverse to reach the coronary arteries – this included severe disease in the femoral arteries, the iliac arteries and the aorta. My efforts to get arterial access were punctuated by recurrent episodes of cardiac arrest. To keep the patient alive was difficult enough, and on all these occasions, the patient required CPR and institution of the resuscitation protocol. More than a dozen people were involved at this stage - nurses, technicians, the intensivist and me, all frantically working to save this patient. You may have already identified some similarities in this procedure with what you have read in "Carlos".

With enormous difficulty, I had access to the right femoral artery. I quickly inserted the IABP, but it proved to be of limited benefit as there had been severe damage to the heart muscle and as a result of some other reasons that make IABP less effective. Accessing the other groin was even more challenging as there was even more severe disease on the left side. Eventually, I abandoned this access route and targeted the right radial artery in the patient's wrist. This was also difficult as the pulse was feeble. With persistence, I was ultimately able to place the access sheath.

My problems were not over with this trivial gain. There was significant tortuosity in the arteries that lead to the heart. To overcome this challenge, I had to try multiple catheters to cannulate the coronary arteries. The majority of catheterization procedures can be performed using two catheters – I needed five before I was able to partially cannulate the left coronary artery. A separate catheter is required to maneuver and fit the left and the right coronary arteries. Worse, this was only the diagnostic part of the procedure, the intervention would be similarly challenging.

The patient had dozens of severe and critical narrowing in all three arteries, including a total blockage of the left anterior descending artery. This artery was heavily calcified, a situation that occurs with severe disease and with the deposition of hard calcium in the coronary arteries.

I quickly contacted, Dr. Solomon, our senior cardiac surgeon and explained to him the critical situation of the patient and his dire prognosis. The surgeon expressed his inability to operate on this patient and he cited, and I believe correctly, the reason as simply no chance of success. Besides, it would take at least an hour to get the operating room ready at 1:30 a.m. I informed Dr. Solomon that I will keep him updated. With the surgical option out, I got back to my task.

This now was my complete collection of challenges - a total obstruction of the Left Anterior Descending artery, severe disease in the other arteries, severe calcification, tortuosity of the vessels, and a patient with profound cardiogenic shock, despite IABP placement.

I will explain the details of what continued to unfold. In summary, I was making no headway even though I continued to struggle for an extremely long time During these maneuvers, I had also evaluated the heart muscle, and it was critically impaired as a result of this heart attack and possibly previous injury. We had also learned that the patient was a heavy smoker and an insulin-requiring diabetic.

The original plans of the New Year celebration were long out of my mind.

I contemplated exchanging the IABP for an Impella, but the patient's severe peripheral vascular disease prevented me from doing so. Selecting the right catheters was so difficult that we almost ran out of suitable catheters in our lab. It took me a very long time to cross the total blockage in the Left Anterior Descending artery with a guide wire. The Left Anterior Descending was the culprit problem – my plan was to first open this artery and place a stent in it and to then consider treating the other two arteries.

When a patient has a heart attack, it is the present-day practice to fix only this culprit blockage. When a patient presents with a heart attack and shock, we try to fix the major blockages in the other arteries as well. This provides the patient better chances of survival.

Again, these efforts were slowed with another prolonged CPR during which the guide wire position was lost. It took additional time to reposition the wire.

The technique of coronary angiography ("cath") and PCI ("angioplasty") are similar up to a point after which they diverge. "Cath" or coronary angiography is the diagnostic part and "angioplasty" or PCI, is the therapeutic part where the blockage that is diagnosed during cath is fixed with angioplasty.

I will now attempt to describe these two procedures in laymen terms. Only a very basic explanation should suffice for your purpose of understanding the related issues. I sincerely hope that this explanation is simple enough for you to comprehend.

During angiography, the left and right coronary arteries are individually hooked with a catheter and dye is injected to opacify this blockage. This injection of dye is recorded by pressing a foot pedal. To treat this blockage, a catheter is chosen that is similar in shape to the one during angiography but which has a larger lumen. Under X-Ray guidance, a slim guide wire is threaded across the blockage. Once this is done, again under X-Rays, a balloon catheter is positioned over the area of blockage. This balloon catheter is inflated with a hand held inflation device. Inflation and deflation of the balloon catheter creates an opening in the artery through which blood can now flow. A stent is then positioned in the same way as a balloon by advancing it over the same guide wire, by positioning it under X-Rays and repeating the process of inflating and deflating. The stent is a metal scaffold, mostly of high-grade steel, that is crimped on the balloon – the stent expands as the balloon is inflated. The balloon is then deflated and it is removed, leaving behind the stent that can be further expanded with a larger balloon, at even higher pressure. This secures the stent firmly in the artery. The diameter and length of balloons and stents are calculated mostly by visual estimation. Sometimes, there is no need to pre- dilate a blockage and we can directly stent it, sometimes the blockage is hard and calcified and it requires complex devices to crack open this blockage after which a stent is placed.

This was precisely the situation with our patient. His arteries were "bone" calcified. Not even the smallest diameter balloon would cross this occluded and calcified vessel. During one of the maneuvers to force the balloon catheter through, the forward resistance pushed the guide wire out. This needed to be repositioned again. In between, the patient again needed CPR. With some difficulty, I placed a second additional wire in the same artery and attempted to slide a thin balloon over one of the two wires. Sometimes, this gliding motion helps the situation. However, this technique did not help. I also tried to place a cutting balloon. This is a special balloon that has three fine blades built on the balloon. Inflation of this special, "cutting" balloon can score a dense blockage and then permit stent placement. This cutting balloon came nowhere near the blockage and I abandoned this strategy.

One of the last options was to use a high-speed rotational cutting device, the "Rotablator." This device was not without its problems in this situation, but it was one of the last salvage options. The device requires a complex set up and I told the nurses to begin set up for this device.

Recognizing that I may not be successful in saving the patient's life, I summoned the nursing supervisor and requested her to apprise the family of our struggles. She returned quickly to inform me that the family clearly understood that the patient would not survive.

As the Rotablator was being set up, I reviewed the patient again to see what else could be done. As a part of the resuscitation protocols, the patient's electrolytes had been corrected. A unit of blood had just arrived, and it was being administered to correct the severe blood loss. The anesthesiologist had verified the correct positioning of the breathing tubes; the intensivist was constantly monitoring the status of ventilation machines.

I had now opened the Rotablator guide wire – this wire behaves quite differently from other guide wires and it is more difficult to navigate. It simply would not cross. I asked for the old guide wire and then began the process of placing the old guide wire again and placing another cath. I continued my struggle with numerous catheters and guide wires and failed with all. Eventually, the patient's critical status and profound disease was overwhelming. After his last cardiac arrest that needed almost 20 minutes of chest compressions, I finally made a decision to abort, and I pronounced the patient dead at 2:35 AM.

It had been 4 hours and 35 minutes when I walked back to the physician's lounge. Kabir had fallen asleep, and Shoba was anxiously pacing the room. 2014 was gone and 2015 had gradually crept in. There was going to be no New Year's celebration for the Mehta family.

Dr. Mehta had been humbled.

CHAPTER 6. CHECKLIST // PREPARING FOR A HEART ATTACK... AND SURVIVING IT

Winter is a season of recovery and preparation
Paul Theroux

I have now reached roughly the midpoint of this book. By careful intent, I had planned to first introduce the concepts of heart attack treatment by illustrating numerous real patients. I assumed that this would provide you with a basic knowledge and a platform before discussing the very specific recommendations for you. I believe we have reached that stage now.

The table on the next page is your checklist of items in "Preparing for a Heart Attack... and Surviving It."

These ten entries on the checklist have taken me a decade to construct in my mind! I used two dogged criteria in preparing this list: 1) each item should provide a personalized recommendation for you; 2) it must be unique – at least from my point of view, it should not have been published before.

I will go into great detail into discussing each element of this list. It is now your responsibility, with the knowledge that you have already accumulated, to master the essence of each of these ten items. I have also placed them in my list of priority with the first item being of the highest importance.

I remain extremely mindful of two practical matters as it relates to our discussion.

Firstly, bookstores, both retail and online, are inundated with numerous materials on treating heart attacks. However, I earnestly believe that my work is exclusive as it actually extracts knowledge from real patients. I also hope that at the conclusion of this book, you will actually start relating your own situation to that of one of the patients.

Not only have I selected the most dramatic and fascinating patients, I have also chosen them specifically to target certain demographics. It is very likely that you will fit within one of the four major groups – males, females, diabetics, and the elderly.

Of course, there is going to be overlap, but there is a scientific reason for my choosing these four groups. Allow me to explain. Symptoms of a heart attack in men and women can be radically different. As I described before, diabetics do not demonstrate classical chest pain. The elderly can be confusing in their clinical presentation of a heart attack. In addition to selecting these four groups, I have purposefully selected more than one patient case for each group – this is to emphasize points that you will benefit from.

The second important issue relates to this book providing you with a guide to help yourself.

This book is not a substitute for a doctor.

Neither is it a source for you to confront your doctor.

Your personal physician, or your cardiologist, knows you and your clinical history the best. Beyond the dictums of this book, you must follow the advice and recommendations of your own physician.

Having stated the above, I remain completely convinced that the knowledge provided to you through this book will only advance your learning about this important personal issue, and it will supplement the care provided by the physician. I must add at this juncture that no amount of preparation in saving you from a catastrophic heart attack is overdone.

A heart attack is a deadly occurrence. You may never get a second chance. There is simply no room for error, so let us get it absolutely right.

Here is your checklist.

PREPARING FOR A HEART ATTACK... AND SURVIVING IT
CHECKLIST
1. Keep Aspirin and the Statin drug handy
2. Count your risk factors
3. Know the name and the address of the hospital nearest you that performs heart attack angioplasty
4. Try to find out if your ambulance services transmit the EKG
5. Keep handy a laminated copy of your EKG
6. Plan a scenario of notifying 911, if you are unconscious
7. Discuss with your spouse/loved one all of the above
8. Assess quickly if you are having a heart attack
9. Express this clearly to the 911 operator
10. Be sure the ambulance takes you to the PCI hospital, and not the nearest one

1. Keep Aspirin and the Statin drug handy

I have previously discussed the role of aspirin and how scientists working for Bayer invented this wonder drug. Now that you understand some aspects of the mechanisms that cause a heart attack, you will clearly value this precious life-saving drug. Let us master this and the statin drugs.

Prior to the coronary artery forming an obstructive clot, a sentinel event occurs in the artery. There is a break in the innermost lining of the coronary artery. This lining is extremely thin, and its rupture leads to a dramatic series of swift and deadly events. Although various factors are recognized that contribute to the rupture of this intimal lining, we   still have not been able to find definite ways to prevent this deadly phenomenon. Clearly, stresses, unusual physical activity, early morning hours, and even cold are known to precipitate heart attacks.

You will now understand the classic description of the person shoveling snow in the morning who has a heart attack.

Breaking of the protective intimal lining exposes a sticky surface for the blood cells and platelets, which precipitously deposit on the exposed surface of the artery after this protective lining has been damaged. The factors that contribute to the rupture of the intimal lining also increase the stickiness of the platelets.

With this crescendo pattern, in a matter of minutes, there is both a breach of the previously healthy lining, and formation of a blood clot. This initial clot can quickly enlarge and become occlusive and result in a heart attack.

The body has numerous counter mechanisms that prevent the formation and propagation of this clot. On the other hand, clotting is also required to stop bleeding. Our body constantly maintains this natural balance – of both forming a clot to stop bleeding and preventing a clot that can cause a heart attack. Various mechanisms in the body contribute to maintaining this healthy equilibrium. The patient's heart rate and blood pressure are important factors in preserving this balance. High glucose levels tilt the balance towards an injurious thrombus. Perhaps the biggest insult that promotes the development of this deadly blood clot is smoking.

As a result of the imbalance in the body's mechanisms, the symptoms leading to a heart attack can be varying. Frequently, patients have crushing chest pain that may somewhat ease. Let us examine this with a previous patient that you have read about. This will make this description easier and provide a better framework for understanding these mechanisms.

Let us review the accountant. You will recall that after he had the initial bout of crushing chest pain, he felt well. This is seen with several

patients who may have a periodic relief in their chest pain. Aspirin is a lifesaver in these situations. It may have been so for Victor too (incidentally, it is recommended to chew the aspirin as that makes it act faster). As Victor felt better, the mechanisms causing the blood clot were interrupted. Sometimes, vigorous heart pumping by itself can dislodge the blood clot or create fissures and fractures through it. This enables blood to trickle down the previously occluded vessel. The outcome mostly depends on the body's natural balance. Some patients will
find relief from their symptoms, whereas others will have a massive heart attack.

The use of aspirin is to precisely create a situation where the formation of this blood clot is either prevented or delayed. Aspirin prevents the activation of these platelets and prevents their deposition on the sticky, denuded arterial surface. It is an absolute lifesaver. Understanding this paragraph and implementing it may give you a second birthday. So please read and understand it well. Aspirin, taken immediately upon recognizing heart attack symptoms, is your best chance to prevent this clot formation and slow its propagation. Although relatively benign, aspirin is not without its risks. In particular, in patients with severely elevated blood pressure, there is a rare possibility of stroke. Some gastrointestinal bleeding can also occur. However, these events are extremely unusual, and the benefits are enormous.

The role of the statin drugs is also important to understand. These drugs are understood to lower the bad, or LDL cholesterol, and increase the good, or HDL cholesterol. It is for this ability of improving the fat ratio that statins are a blockbuster class of drugs. In some ways, we may be overusing these drugs as patients substitute them for improving their diets and increasing exercise. It is all too easy to improve your lipids numbers by taking these drugs. I will discuss this issue later when I discuss about preventing a heart attack.

The statins are not without their hitches. In particular, cramping and muscular fatigue can be debilitating. Several patients end up reducing the dose and quitting these drugs because of these and some other adverse effects.

There is however, another great application of the statins that make them extremely useful during heart attacks. These agents decrease inflammation and stabilize a fatty plaque and prevent its rupture.

In the preceding pages, I discussed how the rupture of the fatty plaque precedes a heart attack. We do not fully understand all mechanisms that cause this rupture. But one of the prevailing scientific theories is that the rupture of the plaque and the intima occurs as a result of ongoing inflammation. Statins, in addition to their protective role of lowering lipids, help in the management of early stages of a heart attack by reducing the inflammation and stabilizing the plaque.

The dose of these two drugs is also an important issue. For the purpose of preventing the heart attack and for the very early management, a full 325mg tablet of aspirin is recommended. This may be available as a single tablet or four 81mg tablets. As explained above, chewable aspirin works faster. The dose of statins and the type of statin do not point to a clear single answer. Several may be used for this purpose; either Lipitor 40 mg or Crestor 10 mg are adequate for this purpose.

2. Count your risk factors

The traditional four big coronary artery disease risk factors include diabetes, smoking, high blood pressure, and elevated lipids. To this, additional factors of the male sex, stress, family history, and middle age should be considered. Beyond this list, a few other scientific factors have also been researched, but their relevance to our topic is more academic than practical.

Let us first concentrate on the big four – these are not too big to fall!

Diabetes, as explained previously in this book, is of two major types. In the more malignant variety, there is a complete lack of insulin in the body (Insulin Dependent Diabetes Mellitus or IDDM) that leads to dangerously high levels of blood glucose. Insulin is a hormone produced by the pancreas that regulates the level of blood glucose. High levels of blood glucose are destructive to numerous organs of the body including the heart, the blood vessels, the kidneys, and even the eyes. Treatment of this severe form of diabetes is by using of insulin that may be administered in a variety of different ways. The less severe form of diabetes is known as non-insulin dependent diabetes mellitus or NIDDM. This type of diabetes can be treated with oral anti-diabetic agents. Although, this is also a severe disease, this type of diabetes is clearly less lethal than the insulin- dependent type. As it relates to coronary artery disease, diabetes causes deposition of fat in the coronary arteries and even contributes to the rupture of the protective plaque. Treatment of both forms of diabetes is essential for the management of coronary artery disease. In our checklist, to know if one is a diabetic is critical. Most of you will clearly know if you suffer from diabetes. The intent of this book is not to create panic. If you are healthy and doing well, you really do not need to run to find out if you are diabetic, but at some stage, this is valuable information about your health that you should correctly know. However, if you are diabetic, the presence of chest pain, whether typical or atypical, is of enormous importance.

The next important risk factor of coronary artery disease is smoking. Smoking is calculated by smoking pack years, which is the number of packs of cigarettes smoked per day multiplied by the years of smoking.

For example, a person who smokes a pack a day for 20 years has a 20-pack year history. Another patient who has smoked half a packet for the last 10 years has 5-pack year history. Clearly, the first patient has had more damage due to the greater amount of tobacco use. Tobacco, smoked through cigarettes and cigars, or chewed, is a source of nicotine, which is extremely injurious to the coronary arteries. Particularly, as it relates to our discussion of heart attacks, nicotine strips the protective lining of the arteries and activates the platelets. It is a most potent accelerator of a heart attack. The good news is that cessation of smoking can virtually eliminate your risk. It is well known that cessation of smoking for up to a year can lower the risk from the insults of nicotine use.

The third risk factor is high blood pressure. The precise numbers that define high blood pressure has been modified periodically. A blood pressure reading has two numbers – the systolic, or the upper value, and the diastolic, or the lower value. Both are important. A persistent elevation of blood pressure more than 130/85 mmHg (millimeters of Mercury, the established scientific unit of this measurement) is considered high blood pressure. As it pertains to our discussion in counting as a risk factor, a controlled blood pressure through medication reduces the risk of a heart attack.

The last of our major risk factors is elevated levels of lipids in the blood. Lipids are basically of two types – blood triglycerides and blood cholesterol. Although both are detrimental and constitute risk factors, cholesterol level is relatively more important. Within cholesterol are two important groups that deserve understanding. A third academic intermediate group requires much more advanced knowledge, and I will not discuss that. The two important cholesterol groups for our comprehension are the good cholesterol or the HDL, and the bad cholesterol, or LDL. HDL is very protective for coronary arteries and it prevents the deposition of fat in the coronary arteries. Significantly, it can be increased with exercise and with the use of statin drugs. As opposed to this, the bad cholesterol, or LDL, is detrimental and it is a potent cause for fat deposition in the coronary arteries.   An LDL level above 130 and an HDL level of below 60 constitutes coronary artery disease risk factors.

Beyond the four major risk factors of diabetes, smoking, high blood pressure, and high lipids, let us briefly understand some other important risk factors.

A positive family history of coronary heart disease constitutes a near relative, a parent, or a sibling, that has suffered a heart attack. Stress, acting through a variety of adverse mechanisms, is also a big contributing factor. You, as has been demonstrated in the clinical presentation of several case studies in this book, already recognize being a middle-aged male, as a risk factor. When taking a look at these lesser risk factors, the one that can be clearly controlled is stress. It is too late to dent family history or our own age and sex!

Having discussed these risk factors, how exactly do they relate to our bucket list? How do they advance our understanding on a day-to-day basis if we are confronted with a heart attack? Let me try to explain.

The more risk factors that you have, the higher is your risk for having a heart attack.

I am sure this was no news to you, and that you had already surmised as much or had read about it. A search on the internet will reveal many risk factor calculators for coronary artery disease and heart attack. I am not going to burden you with a new scheme of calculating, but I want to teach you about the clinical relevance of these factors.

At this stage, let us grasp the various causes of chest pain. I want you to think intelligently for a moment and appraise the anatomy of structures in and around the chest wall. Chest pain can originate from any of these sources. It can come from the chest wall itself, where the rib cage and muscles are located. Chest pain, can, of course, arise from various clinical conditions of the heart. Various lung conditions can also cause chest pain. To make you understand a little more, the heart is located inside the chest wall cavity and the two lungs surround it. Both the heart and the lung have their own special coverings.

The covering around the heart is known as the pericardium, and the one around the lung is known as the pleural lining. Inflammation of either of these protective linings can also cause chest pain. The next organ in the chest cavity to consider is the food pipe and the stomach – this we have already discussed, and we understand how various problems of the stomach and esophagus, can cause chest pain.

Beyond these anatomical structures, anxiety can mimic or worsen symptoms originating from all these organs.

Of course, an entire textbook can be written about the various clinical entities that can cause chest pain from these bodily structures. I will try to discuss the more common reasons that cause chest pain. If you are able to comprehend the bigger and more common causes, differentiating a non-cardiac chest pain from one that causes a heart attack may not be that difficult. It is my endeavor to simplify this for you.

I must emphasize again that none of this acquired knowledge is a substitute of the suggestions made by your own doctor.

Victor, the Accountant, felt his chest pain was from reflux esophagitis. We also understand this an important cause of chest pain. Symptoms of reflux can be very similar to those of a heart attack. The two simple observations that point to reflux disease, also known as GERD (gastrointestinal reflux disease), are its previous occurrence and the ingestion of corrosive foods and beverages. Consuming a few tequilas and spicy Mexican food and then having chest pain, is more likely a result of reflux than of a heart attack. This is common sense deduction; nothing that requires specialized cardiology training.

Two other larger conditions need special mention and understanding. The first pertains to the respiratory system and to the lungs. Lung infections, including attacks of flu, pneumonia, and even asthma can cause chest pain from lung disease. Similarly, viral and bacterial infections can involve the pericardial lining and cause a condition known as pericarditis. The lung and heart infections can present in fashions very similar to a heart attack. Once again, a history of fever, body aches, and weakness will often accompany an infection as opposed to the suddenness of a heart attack. A last condition that can be very confusing, as it causes both chest pain and anxiety is the congenital condition of the mitral valve prolapse. This is seen more commonly in young women.

I can understand that some of this must be confusing. I will simplify these for you and connect the dots in the next few paragraphs. With that, all this medical jargon will quickly become relevant to you.

These various causes of chest pain assume a totally different significance in the presence of risk factors for heart attacks.

See how easily this will now fall into place now!

Chest pain, from any of these conditions, in the presence of risk factors has a higher likelihood of resulting from a heart attack. Conversely, any of these conditions that cause chest pain, in the absence of risk factors, are not a likely to be a heart attack. Now you understand the significance of risk factors and why I went into great detail to help you understand and appreciate their relevance.

Another important confusing entity is muscular pain, particularly an entity known as costochondritis. This condition results from an inflammation of the junction between the rib cage and the sternum bone. This may result from arthritis, muscular injury, and infection after surgery. The chest pain from costochondritis may be minimal or extremely severe, and it can be very frightening, and mimic a heart attack. An easy hint of its occurrence is pronounced tenderness over the chest wall area. Besides, a careful clinical history of recent injury, heavy weight lifting, trauma, recent surgery, or long-standing arthritis all point to costochondritis as a cause of chest pain.

Stress and anxiety can mimic heart attack in numerous ways. It can sometimes become difficult to distinguish anxiety with chest pain from heart attack as a heart attack also presents with symptoms of anxiety.

If you are 48 (Carlos), or 54 (George), or 63 (Victor) – all middle-aged men and smokers, your chest pain may indeed be a heart attack.

Now you may understand my logic of going into great detail when I described these three patients.

If you add other risk factors, such as diabetes, high blood pressure, and high lipids, the chances of the chest pain being a heart attack are increased. It is commonly recognized that two or more risk factors denote a significantly increased chance that the chest pain could be from a heart attack. Several subsequent chapters will help you recognize the very specific presentation of chest pain. As an example, chest pain with difficulty of breathing and causing nausea and sweating is very suggestive of a heart attack.

So far, as it pertains to the risk factors, here is the great news. If you do not have risk factors, then the chest pain is less likely to be a heart attack.

My wife sometimes complains of chest pain that she describes as "I'm having a heart attack!"

But I know that she has no risk factors, whatsoever. Is this a completely safe deduction? Probably not.

In medicine, we never claim to be 100% certain, but I have been correct all the time when my wife complained of chest pain. Of course, I did not ignore her complaints, but it was reassuring because of the simple observation that as she does not have any risk factor, the likelihood of a heart attack is low.

There are a few rare conditions where heart attacks can occur in an absence of risk factors; however, these are extremely uncommon. Let us therefore begin with an accurate analysis of your individual risk factors for a heart attack. Please go ahead right now and establish your individual risk. Assess your risk factors.

If you have coronary artery disease risk factors, mainly smoking, diabetes, high blood pressure, and high lipids, the presence of chest pain should make you seek immediate help and call 9-1-1.

Of course, you can be wrong and indeed you may not be having a heart attack. Count this as a blessing. But, this is not a situation where you want to be wrong.

Let us extend this knowledge further and make some important deductions - the more risk factors you have, the higher is the likelihood that the chest pain is from a heart attack. This should immediately alert you, and it may be the time to take aspirin and call 9-1-1.

Now, let us examine the reverse. Chest pain, with no risk factors, gives you time to pause and reflect, whether non-cardiac factors may be at play.

Beyond everything I have informed you, you will never be wrong by calling 9-1-1, if, and whenever, you have a doubt.

3. Know the name and the address of the hospital nearest you that performs heart attack angioplasty

This issue is novel, and its search can make some people very upset. This is not a stricture that patients traditionally seek; yet it is a matter of paramount importance so far as a heart attack is concerned. I strongly believe that this information should be voluntarily made available by individual hospitals, and that it should be available in the public domain. It is your right, as a taxpayer, to know and to assess your local hospital's ability to treat heart attacks. I consider this as your fundamental right.

This is an important and provocative discussion.

A killer heart attack is very different from an elective situation where you may seek advice from friends, relatives, your doctor, and the media for the best facility to treat you. In the catastrophic emergency of a heart attack, your options are severely limited.

I am convinced that as the public awareness of this topic increases, it will improve the performance of hospitals that perform primary angioplasty. In addition, the process of how a patient with a heart attack reaches the hospital will improve too.

Therefore, the time for you to seek out this information is now.

A few years ago, I was lecturing in Dubai, on this topic. I emphasized the urgency of treating heart attack by sharing a poignant observation. I stated that the heart attack requires immediate local treatment, and that wealthy Arabs, who seek out the Mayo and the Cleveland Clinic for elective treatment, need a skilled facility to treat their heart attack. Going to the Cleveland Clinic when having a heart attack, is not an option, for even the wealthiest.

The situation for you, my readers, is the same. You need, as a taxpaying citizen, to demand excellent 24/7 heart attack treatment in your local community. Begin this process by knowing which hospitals provide this service.

4. Try to find out if your ambulance services transmit the EKG

This issue is even more contentious. However, its knowledge is as important as that of item number 3. Again, you have a right to demand superior services. You paid for these, so you might as well demand excellence. As I have illustrated to you through numerous case studies in this book, pre-hospital management of a heart attack can be life- saving. Every minute is precious. The entire STEMI process can be significantly improved by making the most accurate diagnosis, and, if possible, bypassing the emergency room. However, this can occur only after there is increased accuracy in diagnosis of the EKG that the paramedics have performed. To increase the accuracy of the diagnosis, there are two pathways. The first is to exhaustively train our paramedics. The second choice is to incorporate

EKG transmission capability into our ambulances.

Will your tax district jump onboard and start investing in transmission technology in their ambulances? Not likely, as things presently stand. But if public demand for this service is vociferous, then this necessary change will occur. I am convinced that this service should be demanded from our local EMS service.

5. Keep handy a laminated copy of your EKG

Knowledge about the importance of EKG record keeping can be extremely helpful. Many clinical conditions mimic a heart attack on an EKG. A comparison with the previous EKG can facilitate the correct diagnosis. If you have had a previous EKG, it is a good idea to keep handy a laminated copy, or even better, a digital version that is readily available. Should you be unfortunate to have chest pain, a readily available previous EKG that can be compared to the present one, can be enormously beneficial. It may also be a good idea, in particular, if you have risk factors for coronary artery disease, to obtain an EKG at your convenience, and keep a copy of it. This is relatively easy to obtain – it is inexpensive and widely available.

6. Plan a scenario of notifying 911 if you are unconscious

Since heart attacks can cause unconsciousness, I have mentioned this scenario. This situation is similar to your having a living will. Discussing heart attack treatment options should become an important topic between children and grandchildren when they are caring for their elderly relatives. Various medical alert devices can be useful and searching for these is a worthwhile endeavor.

7. Discuss with your spouse/loved one all the above

This is an extension of number 6 and it is self-explanatory.

8. Assess quickly if you are having a heart attack

On the basis of everything that I have attempted to teach, you should now be able to ascertain with a high degree of accuracy if you are having a heart attack. In the preface of this book, I stated that I have performed primary PCI on three cardiologists who had neglected their symptoms. Self-denial is a dangerous exercise when confronted with chest pain. Many patients die as they fall into this track of self-denial. Remember how Victor almost talked himself and his wife Grace into proceeding to see the baseball game in Cincinnati. This is a very common occurrence. The chest pain interrupts our planned activity. This could be as simple as reporting to work, or more demanding such as a court appearance. It could be in pursuit of long-planned leisure activity such as going on vacation or on a cruise.

Many of us are bigger risk takers, and this has been a practiced art in our lives. This particular group is especially vulnerable to self-denial.

It is quite normal and understandable how wishful thinking immediately and completely overcomes intellect. The knowledge I have tried to impart to you about the life- threatening dangers of heart attack should overwhelm your self-denial. Wishful thinking and self-denial are terrible gambles if and when you are confronted with a heart attack. You will always lose in the casino where you are wagering your life for self-denial.

The role of an intelligent life partner in these critical situations is extremely important. Remember Briana and Grace. They immediately squashed self-denial and wishful thinking and sought immediate care for their loved ones.

You will never lose by spending a few hours in an emergency room if you are wrong. More importantly, if you resist the temptation to self-deny, and your chest pain is indeed a heart attack, then you will thank me forever for raising your awareness on this very important observation.

To this aspect of self-denial, I must add urgency. Not only should self-denial not factor into your intellect, you should make a very speedy decision and call 9-1-1.

Of course, this traumatic event will mess up your day and it will be enormously disruptive. But it may save your life and enable you to live healthy without heart damage. This is, in a sense, "preparing for a heart attack… and surviving it." You prepare by understanding that you will not self-deny and think wishfully as a result of the intellectual gain from this book. In this way, you will survive the heart attack.

9. Express clearly to the 911 Operator, "I think I am having a heart attack"

As a result of what you have learned and from your quick inference that you may be having a heart attack, express it so to the 911 operators. The response mechanism for heart attacks can be different in various communities. Often, specialized ambulances are sent for heart attacks and even the paramedics may be better equipped and trained.

10. Be sure the ambulance takes you to this hospital, and not the nearest one

As I have discussed in various parts of this book, a heart attack patient receives a STEMI intervention at hospitals that provide this service. By ending up at a non-PCI facility, you are instituting huge delays that may be detrimental to your care. In addition, the smaller hospitals may begin treatment with thrombolytic agents, or clot busters. This complicates the situation completely and your overall success may be lowered. Although it is now a norm for a heart attack patient to be taken to a primary PCI hospital, this cannot be taken for granted. You may not need to over-emphasize this point. Yet this is critical, its importance paramount, and this knowledge will ensure your access in a heart attack to the appropriate facility.

In helping you prepare for a heart attack, and survive it, the above-described checklist is being made available for you to detach and post in a handy   place.

CHAPTER 7. MARY AND ANNA – HEART ATTACKS IN WOMEN

It may be the cock that crows, but it is the hen that lays the eggs.
Margaret Thatcher

July 19th, 2014 will remain a memorable day for Mary and Anna.

It was going to be an exhausting day. Mary Stuart had begun the day in earnest. Most mornings, she awoke at 6:45. She made coffee and scanned her emails. Business had been stressful recently. Her flower distributors from Colombia had demanded an unprecedented 15% price increase citing the weakness in the Colombian peso. The negotiations with an alternative supplier from Ecuador were not fruitful. Sales were stagnant for the last three months and 10% down for the year overall. In order to make payroll, she had decided to let go off Lydia, the quality inspector at Worldwide Flowers, the company that Mary had founded 15 years ago. Lydia had been the second employee in the company, which had now grown to 22 employees and that now generated > $ 2 million in annual revenues. However, net income had horribly stalled because of the increasing expenses. At this rate, Mary concluded, that she would need to draw into her line of credit just to make payroll. Letting Lydia go was emotionally taxing. Lydia had been a fine employee and had been widowed three years ago. It was almost like disappointing a family member. This was particularly distressing to Mary. The previous evening, she had discussed this decision with her husband, Frank. Both had concluded that it was the right choice for the company. Worse, additional employees will need to be let go. There was simply no other way. Competition for the business had been increasing, and there was simply no way to increase prices. Where Frank and Mary differed was how to inform Lydia. Both had prepared an exit package for Lydia that went beyond the employee agreement. Both, the firm's accountant, and Frank's cousin, George, who did part-time legal work for the company, had signed off on the retirement package for Lydia. Frank felt that Joan Meyers, the general manager, should inform Lydia of the company decision.

However, Mary had decided that she would do this herself, that morning.

Much else needed to be done.

By the afternoon, Frank and Mary had to make a final decision on the venue site for their daughter Maria's wedding. The final decision lay between having the wedding at the swanky, new Mandarin Oriental Hotel in lovely Brickell Key or at the magnificent Renaissance Villa, Vizcaya. The latter was clearly the nicer option; it was much more expensive, but it's fantastic location and prestige were worth it. The big snag, however, was the limited number of private contractors that Vizcaya permitted for the various event items. Both Frank and Mary were not satisfied with this arrangement, and they especially did not like the menus that had been suggested.

As these thoughts dispersed in Mary's mind, the phone rang. It showed an unknown caller. Irrespective, Mary answered – it was, after all, the instinct of a mother who had raised two children. It turned out to be her son, Frank Jr., calling from Philadelphia. It was not good news. Junior had been misbehaving again. He was fumbling with his story, and Mary knew that this was going to be another long exercise to extract the truth. According to Junior, he had returned around midnight to his dorm from a birthday party for Claire, his girlfriend. When he woke this morning, he could not find his phone. This was his roommate's phone that he was using to call his mother. Mary knew right away, that this was at best, only partially truthful and she was furious. This was the third phone in a year that Junior had lost. The second one was when he jumped into the swimming pool with the phone in his back pocket. It was simply nauseating.

"How much did you drink?" she demanded.

"A few beers," retorted Junior.

"How many?" she insisted.

"A few," Junior shot back in an accusatory tone.

This was not a good conversation, and particularly not at this moment, when Mary had a hundred more important things on her mind.

Frank had been hearing this conversation, and he motioned Mary to pass him the phone, for him to take care of the problem. But Mary knew better. She knew that Frank would give into their son's nonsense, and find him an alternative phone, instead of getting to the bottom of the problem. However, this had gone on for too long and Junior's recklessness was out of control. His grades had been falling; he had been drinking much more than he admitted. Claire, Junior's new girlfriend also irked Mary. Beyond the exorbitant tuition and the expensive boarding, Frank and Mary had been sending Junior several additional payments by Quick Pay. This morning's incidence with Junior would mean the purchase of another iPhone. She wanted to put her foot down and ground Junior. Worse, he now admitted that the "few beers" were eight. This made Mary even more furious. Junior also admitted that he may have recollected it wrong and that it was closer to 3 a.m. when he returned to the dorm. He had absolutely no recollection how the phone was lost.

Just when this call had degenerated into yelling, the house phone rang.

It was the gardener, Jorge, announcing he could not come on Friday. This was a disaster. Mary's parents were driving from North Carolina, and the yard looked terrible.

This is crazy.

Who should she continue to talk to on the phone - the gardener, who was canceling on her, or her impossible son?

Of course, she made the right decision and informed Jorge that she would call him back later. It was more important to settle this drinking issue. She was distressed to no end. It was not only a few beers; hard liquor was also involved. How does a phone disappear after drinking a few beers? As a mother, she knew that this was clearly worse, but there was no way that Junior was admitting or mending his ways.

Junior was so different from their sweet daughter, Maria, a top student, on a college scholarship, who was a kind and gentle soul. Maria had just been accepted into NYU School of Nursing, that she planned to join after her wedding to her sweetheart, Jason. Everything was looking up for this young couple.

Why could Junior not learn from Maria? Everything with him was a problem. Frank and Mary had alternated between being generously giving to borderline hostile, but nothing was working, like on this morning.

Frank yanked the phone from Mary and yelled even more at Junior.

This was not going to go anywhere. Mary was intensely frustrated. Shaking her head, she walked to the kitchen to get a glass of water. It was 8:30 already, and she was going to meet Lydia at 10. In between, she needed to stop at Wells Fargo Bank and discuss the Line of Credit with the Bank Manager.

"This is insane. I can't take it anymore." She concluded as she sank into the sofa and sipped water.

Suddenly, something else was not right.

She felt dizzy. She placed her left hand on her brow and paused, feeling like she was going to faint.

"This child is going to kill me," she raged. Brushing off her uneasiness, she went back to the kitchen where the conversation between father and son had degenerated. She took the phone back from Frank. She now addressed Junior more calmly. She informed Junior that after the last time when he had lost his phone, she had bought additional insurance that would now come in handy. Having stated this, Mary lamented her profound disgust and she again implored Junior to get his life together. With this, she thought she was done. But this child was impossible. He demanded another $250 for an assortment of new expenses. Another argument resulted from this outrageous demand. Somehow peace descended on the Stuart home when Mary compromised by agreeing to wire $150 to Junior.

By this time, Mary felt clearly unwell.

She was distinctly dizzy, and she was also sweating. Frank remarked that she looked pale. "This is what Junior has done to us," she retorted as she walked away to take a quick shower.

In the few minutes when Mary took a quick shower, the feeling of being unwell persisted. There was lightheadedness and Mary felt off balance. These symptoms persisted as Mary drove to meet the Bank Manager. To make matters worse, the meeting with the manager was protracted. The Assistant Manager needed to be brought in, and lengthy discussions ensued as the managers explained the new lending policies at the bank.

Mary called her office to push her meeting with Lydia to after lunch.

Discussions with the bankers continued - all along, Mary continued to feel unwell. She now felt aching in both shoulders. She felt nauseated and also noticed a vague abdominal discomfort.

Something was not right.

Was she getting the flu?

Or, were the events of that day simply overwhelming?

Clearly it was the latter, she concluded, as Lydia walked into the room for the difficult exit interview.

Lydia was inconsolable. As Mary got up to hug Lydia and comfort her, she fainted. Lydia steadied her fall and yelled out for help. Mary was now awake but very unwell. Lydia took her to the bathroom where Mary vomited. She was pale, dizzy and her shoulders ached with severe pain. Lydia kept apologizing for this situation and told Mary to relax. It was all intensely chaotic.

Mary yelled out, "I need to see my doctor!"

Nancy, the secretary, called Dr. Gonzales. The doctor was making rounds at the hospital, and his staff informed that they would try to reach the doctor. It was early afternoon, and Mary had now been unwell for more than 4 hours.

A few miles across town, in Hialeah, this Tuesday morning was joyfully unfolding for Anna. Her husband, Victor, 65, a manager at Publix Supermarket, had left for work at the usual time. After Victor left, Anna did a few chores in the house before their daughter Maria, rang the bell to drop off their granddaughter, Annabelle, before Maria went to work.

This had been a fantastic time in Anna's life. She had gladly volunteered to take care of her granddaughter as Maria went to work. This had worked out beautifully. Each morning, Monday to Thursday, Maria would drop off Annabelle at 9:30 and return to pick her up at 3:30. No daycare was needed, and Maria was at complete peace with the knowledge that Annabelle was in the safe custody of her mother.

Annabelle was an adorable child. Anna identified so much of Maria in her granddaughter. Today was another happy day for her. Strapping Annabelle in her stroller, Anna threw the baby bag on her shoulder. Both left for a merry morning in the park.

As Anna pushed the stroller, she felt a strange discomfort in her chest. Suddenly, her heart was racing. She had never experienced this before. Her breathing became heavy, and she decided to sit down on the first bench, as they entered the park. By this time, Anna was visibly unwell. The chest pressure was more pronounced, and there was severe pain in her jaw. The palpitations were persistent, and she felt unusually fatigued. She rubbed her chest and tried to take a few deep breaths as she thought about what to do. She clearly felt unwell, but "this will pass," she surmised.

Annabelle had been happily chirping throughout. For Anna, these were, as always, beautiful sounds. Perhaps, as a result of this bliss, within a few minutes, her breathing got better, and the chest discomfort had eased. It still appeared safer to return home. This time around, Anna pushed the stroller a little more gently, as she walked more cautiously back to her home. With some difficulty, Anna reached home. She wanted to call Maria and speak to her, but "I should be okay in the house," she concluded. It was time to feed Annabelle, and she did so joyfully. However, the feeling of being unwell was persistent, and Anna was concerned. It was about noon, and the baby fell off to sleep. So, did Anna.

In the Coconut Grove offices of Worldwide Flowers, pandemonium was unfolding. A trusted employee had been fired; business was dull; and the owner had just fainted. Joan Meyers, Mary Stuart's manager had offered to drive Mary to Dr. Gonzales' office after the doctor returned their call.

The doctor's office was frenzied. Apparently, the physician's assistant had taken a day off, and the office was short-staffed. The receptionist, who knew Mary, quickly took her to the doctor's office. Within 5 minutes, Dr. Gonzales was with her.

The doctor had aged, Mary thought as she glanced at him. She had been his patient for almost 15 years, and she trusted his judgment. The doctor was alarmed, as Mary looked very uncomfortable. He instantly made a brilliant decision that would prove to be life-saving. He asked Joann, his nurse, to immediately perform an EKG.

At 2:37 p.m., Mary Stuart's life changed. She was having a massive heart attack! As Dr. Gonzales saw the massive ST-segment elevation on the EKG, he pulled a chair next to Mary, who was lying on the examining table. Calmly, he told her, "Mary, I know this will shock you, but you are having a heart attack. And there is no doubt about it."

Mary was shocked. "How could this be? Me? Having a heart

attack?" She shook her head in disbelief.

"I will explain all of this, but I must first make some urgent phone calls." Dr. Gonzales told Mary. Instructing Joann to stay with Mary, he rushed out.

His office was 10 minutes away from Gateway Hospital. He knew that Mary needed an angioplasty, but he had no idea how this would occur. It seemed best to call 9-1-1 and safely transport her. Should he place an intravenous? No, that can wait. Mary was stable. He should give her an aspirin. He yelled for his front desk staff to call 9-1-1, as he retraced his steps to the examining room. Mary was calmer, and on the phone with Frank, who was equally shocked. Joann easily spotted the bare box containing aspirin amongst the assortment of drug samples in the office closet. Quickly, Dr. Gonzales poured out 4 mini Aspirin tablets that Mary swallowed with a gulp of water. Dr. Gonzales rushed back to the front desk where the staff informed him that the ambulance would arrive in 10 minutes. His office now had Dr. Nathan, the ER physician at Gateway Hospital, on the phone line. Dr. Gonzales told Dr. Nathan that there was pronounced ST-elevation in leads II, III, AVF, and that he was faxing the EKG over. Dr. Nathan inquired if they had connected a portable monitor to the patient. The office did not have one. Dr. Gonzales provided Dr. Nathan with a quick medical history on Mary - that she had borderline high blood pressure, borderline diabetes, and elevated cholesterol, for which she was being treated with Lipitor. Dr. Nathan inquired about the intensity of chest pain and Dr. Gonzales replied that there was none. He informed that the blood pressure was 100/60, and the patient was complaining of marked dizziness and stomach pains. Dr. Nathan requested Dr. Gonzales to stay with the patient until the paramedics arrived. Dr. Nathan informed Dr. Gonzales that he was going to notify the cath lab for a possible STEMI intervention.

The paramedics arrived sooner than the ETA of 10 minutes. They performed another EKG that was very similar to the one performed by Dr. Gonzales. Mary was quickly connected to a monitor, and the ambulance sped away to the emergency room. At the ER, the registration could not be completed as Mary did not have her United Healthcare Insurance Card with her. However, Dr. Gonzales' office was sending this information over. After a short stop in the ER, where Dr. Nathan evaluated Mary, she was rushed to the cath lab, where she arrived at 3:31p.m.

At Anna's home, there was controlled disarray. Maria had arrived and was shocked to see her mother whose condition, by this time, had noticeably deteriorated. She was in horrible pain and the chest pressure had become worse. There was more difficulty in breathing, and she could barely stand. Maria knew that something was terribly wrong. Holding Annabelle in her arms, she made a quick decision to call 9-1-1: this brilliant decision saved her mother's life. About 10 minutes later, the EKG performed by the paramedics, showed that Anna was having "a massive heart attack."

I had responded to the first STEMI call for Mary Stuart, a 51-year-old female with a massive inferior wall MI. I confronted a confused patient and a frightened husband as I rushed to the cath lab. Frank exclaimed, "She had no symptoms of a heart attack!" I quickly replied that women often presented in this fashion, and that I would explain this in detail after helping his wife. As the cath lab technicians were prepping Mary, the nurse, Amy, sedated her and reassured her. Primarily, Mary kept questioning how this could be happening to her. Her angioplasty was straightforward, 100% occluded right coronary artery that was easily stented after extracting the blood clot with an Export catheter. The result of opening the occluded artery was perfect although the left ventricle was mildly sluggish. With time, I told both Mary and Frank later, there was every possibility that this would recover because the angioplasty had rapidly restored blood to the heart muscle. Explaining to them about the "atypical presentation" was a little more difficult, as it also got interrupted by a STEMI call from the hospital operators. It was for Anna, the 64-year-old Hispanic grandmother, who had a massive anterior wall myocardial infarction. At 4:08 p.m., she had arrived at the emergency room. By 4:32 p.m., I had already stented her 95% occluded left anterior descending coronary artery. This was also an easy procedure. The heart muscle was completely normal.

Anna had been troubled with only one question, "Is Annabelle with Maria?"

The case descriptions of Mary Stuart and Anna Rodriguez are the "atypical presentation" for women when they are having a heart attack.

In the SINCERE database, 38% of the patients have been women that had a mean age of 68. These are important statistics when comparing to the mean age for men of 59. In our country, a heart attack occurs every 48 seconds. Women must not feel immune to heart attacks. In fact, most studies demonstrate that women have worse outcomes with heart attack than men. A study analyzing more than 400,000 heart attacks, published this week, suggest that the outcomes for women are much worse than previously estimated.

Let us educate ourselves more about women and heart attacks. It is the "atypical presentation" of heart attack in women that makes the situation much more difficult. The symptoms of crushing, mid sternal chest pain, and a feeling of an elephant sitting on the chest are missing. These classical symptoms, experienced by men when having heart attacks, are completely absent in most women who present with heart attacks. The symptoms can be very vague. There is a feeling of being unwell, of something not being right. The chest pain is also more ambiguous, and it is vaguely located. More commonly, the symptoms are of nausea, palpitations, unusual fatigue, chest pressure, joint pain, pain in arms, sweating, and feelings of lightheadedness and dizziness. When compared to men that have classic crushing chest pain, the presentation in women can be a diagnostic dilemma. Even more troubling is the fact that these symptoms are often ignored or not taken seriously, definitely not to the same level as they are done for men. This results in women presenting to the hospital or seeking 9-1-1 help much later after their clinical presentation. This troubling statistic probably accounts for the adverse outcomes associated with women when they have heart attacks.

Let us now evaluate what was happening with Mary Stuart and Anna Rodriguez. They were not having the crushing chest pain that was experienced by Victor, the Accountant, and George, the Attorney. These are essential points to understand in this book. In fact, they may represent the biggest learning objective of this book. Mary Stuart did not experience any of the classic symptoms of chest pain, shortness of breath, and profuse sweating. It was left to the brilliance of Dr. Gonzales, the mature and experienced physician, who recognized these atypical symptoms. The doctor, confronting a middle- aged patient with a history of smoking and diabetes, who is complaining of an elephant sitting on top of his chest, and who has profound clamminess and sweating, does not require great wisdom in making an easy diagnosis! But a physician confronting 51-year-old women with borderline risk factors and atypical symptoms, is extremely smart, well-read, and well- versed in taking care of women with a heart attack.

Various personal, social, cultural, financial, and religious factors cloud the judgment of women who are having a heart attack. In my own research, we are exploring the role of these factors in contributing to the worse outcomes in women. This research, Global Lumen Organization of Women (GLOW), is prospectively collecting patient data in 10 developing countries.

There are two other differentiating features - one is an important numerical number to keep in mind. The other relates to delayed presentation when women have a heart attack. The statistic to remember is that women are much older than men when they have a heart attack - women present almost a decade later than men. We have seen this in the SINCERE database. The troubling pattern of delayed presentation occurs because of a variety of reasons.

Let us once again review Mary Stuart and Anna Rodriguez. Mary was initially dismissive of her symptoms, and she did not seek medical attention till almost 4 hours after her heart attack. This may have resulted in the slight damage to her heart muscle. This is a very common occurrence despite Mary's obvious intellect and maturity. The demands of her daily life were simply overwhelming as she juggled her multiple priorities of a mother, a homemaker, and a businesswoman who was experiencing numerous stressful work challenges.

Heart attacks were the domain of men, compounded by stressful work situations. However, men are fortunate that their symptoms are easy to spot. This explains why men present faster with their emergencies. Mary initially dismissed her symptoms because of her frustrations with Junior. Next, the bank managers clouded her thinking. All along, as it happens with men, had she presented with crushing chest pain, her diagnosis may have been simpler and the call for medical attention may have been more urgent. Even during Mary's terrible confrontation with Lydia, whom she had to fire, she ignored her symptoms that had now become more pronounced.

Although these symptoms are "atypical," this pattern is classic of postponing symptoms and delaying the call to emergency care when women have heart attacks.

The kind and gentle, Anna Rodriguez, was simply preoccupied with the responsibilities of taking care of Annabelle. She tolerated fairly severe symptoms and she did not want to burden her daughter Maria. There are numerous personal and cultural undertones, several of which are being researched methodically. It may be a continuation of a pattern of self-sacrifice of both motherhood and grand motherhood that prevented Anna from immediately seeking care.

In my experience of caring for patients with heart attacks in Miami, there are two clear patterns of presentation. The first is an early morning presentation that is consistent with the greater prevalence of heart attacks occurring in the morning. The next group is observed in grandparents who present with heart attacks between 4 and 6 p.m. - often in situations similar to that of Anna Rodriguez.

So, what is the take home message for the readers and what can they assimilate from this chapter? Women are almost as likely as men to have a heart attack. Their symptoms are clearly atypical. They must remain vigilant to their differing physiology, as should their family members. For healthcare providers, including doctors, a far better understanding of these differing characteristics is paramount.

CHAPTER 8. CARING FOR YOUR ELDERLY LOVED ONES

The fear of death follows from the fear of life. A man who lives fully is prepared to die at any time.
Mark Twain

To help my reader understand some difficult issues relating to the elderly, I have compiled the following chapter using three patients whom I treated this year. You may be able to identify your loved one amongst the case histories of these three patients. I urge you to read this chapter carefully, as it will help you prepare to deal with the extreme challenges when your elderly loved one experiences a heart attack.

These issues go beyond the care that is required when an elderly patient is having a heart attack. I genuinely believe that some of these issues will be the hardest you will confront in your life. They may relate to challenges such as to not proceed with angioplasty and accept fate as it unfolds. They may also include decision making for your most beloved person in extremely rushed circumstances when you will be far away and frightened about the prospect of losing your loved one. Of course, these challenges involve issues regarding hospitalization, payments, and the completely altered scenarios of follow- up care after a heart attack.

Writing this chapter has been the hardest task of compiling this book. Addressing these issues has required wisdom and maturity, and it has nothing to do with my interventional cardiology skills. Almost all these observations have been made after caring for several hundred elderly patients who were having heart attacks. In some cases, the Primary Angioplasty was performed for elderly patients that were incompetent and no family was available. In most situations involving medical care of the elderly, physicians often have enough time to make meticulous efforts to reach the family. However, this is totally different when a patient is having a heart attack, and when every minute counts. Often, there are clear, living will directives, which assist with not resuscitating and prolonging life. However, the situation with a heart attack is totally different. Frequently, in 30 minutes, or even less, the heart attack can be aborted and the patient's health can be restored. It is extremely tricky for the interventional cardiologist to manage this situation.

On the other hand, for a truly elderly patient with clearly limited lifespan, death from a heart attack is truly not a bad option. I write the above sentence with extreme sensitivity and with utmost respect for your loved one. I will deal with this difficult issue in more detail after presenting the following cases.

Joyce Grant presented to me on her 89th birthday. Joyce was living alone after the death of her husband, Henry, 11 years earlier. She required part-time assistance with living, which her daughter, Elizabeth, was overseeing. Joyce could still drive, and she enjoyed doing this despite Elizabeth's concerns. A compromise had been reached between Elizabeth and Joyce that allowed Joyce to drive for short distances in the presence of her aide, Patricia. Joyce had been an extremely active real-estate pioneer. She had begun a real-estate management firm 60 years ago that had flourished and that was now managed by Elizabeth. Joyce had a history of mild diabetes, controlled high blood pressure, and mild Parkinsonism that had manifested 5 years ago. She had no problem with her urination or bowel movement. She maintained an excellent appetite and enjoyed watching TV. She had been an excellent golfer, a skilled painter, and an avid hiker. Joyce had one daughter, three grandchildren, and two great grandchildren. Although most of her medical conditions were well controlled, she still carried a surprisingly long list of 13 medications, whose administration alone required a full-time attendant. The day when Joyce had a heart attack was relatively typical for her. Patricia, the aide, had helped her dress. Joyce had decided to drive her Honda Accord to Dr. Jason Smith, the Internist, located a mile away from her home in Coconut Grove. Patricia helped Joyce to her car and kept the walker in the car trunk. Slowly and carefully, Joyce drove off to see Dr. Smith. She crossed Tigertail Avenue and paused at the long traffic light to make left onto US 1. The light changed, but Joyce had stalled. Patricia exclaimed, "Move, Joyce. The Light is green." But Joyce did not respond.

Patricia realized that Joyce had fainted. The car driver in the adjacent lane had recognized this emergency and was alert enough to call 9-1-1. The EMS responded quickly, and they found Joyce to be having a heart attack. They transported her to nearby Bayside Medical Center. Joyce was found to be in heart failure and required placement of a breathing tube – this is called intubation.

Patricia was panicking, as she could not reach Elizabeth on the phone.

The ER physician, Dr. Gupta, was forced to make a critical decision. Both he and I reviewed the situation and recognized the immediate challenges that confronted us: how to care for Joyce, 89-years old, who was having a heart attack, but there was no consent available to treat and manage the heart attack?

Patricia had no other phone number – she knew the number for

Joseph, the grandson, who was "a famous architect in Miami," but she did not know his full name and had left his number at her home. She was trying to call her own daughter to retrieve Joseph's phone number when Dr. Gupta and I approached her. It was obvious that there was no family available, but we needed to make an urgent and life-saving decision that took into consideration the overall condition of the patient.

Of course, both of us were mindful of the legal implications of this situation. Clearly, there was a possibility that Joyce would not survive. On the other hand, the angioplasty could completely abort the heart attack and result in a miraculous save.

But would this have been the patient's decision? Would this also be the decision of the family?

We were losing precious minutes. As we discussed, the skilled Dr. Gupta, took excellent care of Joyce. He asked the nurses to place a Foley catheter for emptying the urinary bladder and for treating the heart failure. He also quickly assessed the status of the breathing machine. Joyce already being intubated had complicated our decision. This, too, had been performed as a life-saving emergency situation.

I will describe my rationale for the decisions I made but let me first complete the clinical story. My cath lab team and the ER nurses quickly transported the patient to the cath lab. I performed a relatively easy angioplasty. This simple procedure completely opened the very large, left anterior descending coronary artery that was causing the heart attack and heart failure. Joyce did extremely well after the procedure. Considering her advanced age, her lung specialist was appropriately cautious in removing her breathing tube too soon. With sensible care that she received from the doctors and nurses, Joyce was able to gradually ambulate, and she left the hospital in a week's time. Elizabeth and Joseph had finally been contacted. They profoundly thanked me after the procedure. I introduced them to Susanna Smith, the hospital social worker, who offered to guide them with the options of Long-term Care.

Here is the real dilemma for the reader: what would have been Elizabeth and Joseph's reaction had Joyce expired during the procedure?

David Cohen was 79, and his wife Norma, 76. Both lived a comfortable retired life in Key Biscayne, Florida. The Cohen's had two children, Samantha and Peter. Samantha worked for the United Nations, and, for the last three years, had been posted in Angola. Peter had a tire manufacturing business based in Canton, Ohio. Neither child was close to their parents. Numerous personal and financial disputes had risen, and it made for a difficult family structure. David and Norma had numerous health conditions. Both had a revolving door pattern in and out of emergency rooms – David for his vicious pulmonary emphysema from his years of smoking and Norma from frequent complications related to her diabetes, high blood pressure, and urinary incontinence. The two had recently converted their Medicare insurance to a local HMO in order to afford the numerous drugs that were needed to treat them.

David and Norma were dining at the Hunan Restaurant in Key Biscayne. An argument had erupted. First, Norma had become livid; now David was the worse one. Both were reacting to the estimate a roofer had given them to repair their roof leak. Their insurance company had refused payment. David felt that he should ask Peter for help. Norma had disagreed. This resulted in the fight. At this stage, David was visibly shaking with anger, and Norma was telling him to calm down or he would have a stroke.

Instead of the stroke, David had a heart attack!

Fortunately for him, his presentation was classic – a severe crushing chest pain with marked difficulty in breathing. He knew that he was having a heart attack, as did Norma. In their numerous hospital visits, they had encountered heart attacks before.

The previous year, their neighbor, Jack, had died at home from a heart attack. Help was called promptly, and the EMS responded fast. David was quickly and safely transported to Bayside Medical Center. Transfer to the cath lab was faultless, and I began the procedure.

Everything else was difficult thereafter, including specific issues you may encounter when your loved one has a heart attack.

David had extremely severe coronary artery disease. Although I treated the right coronary artery, which was totally blocked and the source of the heart attack, this was only partial treatment. In addition to this culprit artery, David had significant additional blockages. It was my opinion that David would require open-heart surgery to bypass these numerous blockages and to give him the best chance of survival. There was a 90% complex occlusion of the left main coronary artery and additional challenging disease both in the left circumflex and in the left anterior descending artery. The heart muscle was already impaired. The successful angioplasty that I performed probably saved David's life, but this was not full resolution of his heart problems. It was clear to me that in a relatively short time David would require open-heart surgery to bypass. To make matters worse, on the second day after treatment of his heart attack, David had further worsening of his heart failure, for which he required insertion of the breathing tube. The heart surgeon, Dr. Ruiz, wanted to operate early, and I concurred.

When we both proposed this scenario to Norma, she freaked out. She simply could not decide. When we suggested that she speak to the family, she was extremely reluctant. She was mainly concerned about who would take care of David after his surgery, as they had no money to pay for long-term care. Dr. Ruiz had an abrupt conversation with Peter, who retorted, "The old man deserved this. He was smoking like a chimney all his life. What else did he expect?" After uttering this volatile response, Peter hung up the phone.

This unfortunate story worsens.

Norma finally consented for surgery and David underwent a long and complicated operation. Not only did his heart failure not improve, he had further kidney failure, and his lungs finally gave out. After 6 agonizing weeks in the hospital, David expired.

Norma remains distraught, and the family tore further apart.

Irma Rodriguez was 97, frail and pale when I saw her, but she was completely alert, remarkably jovial, and a very kind soul. She had been brought to Gateway Hospital from Miami Springs Nursing Home after the nursing aide found her less responsive. Her examination had been especially difficult, as she had been moribund for weeks. Although her overall hygiene appeared acceptable, a closer examination revealed obvious evidence of suboptimal care. Her adult diaper smelled foul; her nails were overgrown, and there was a severe bed sore on the left hip. An intravenous had been started to administer fluids and it had dramatically improved her clinical condition. This was probably because Irma had been dehydrated. A routine EKG demonstrated a fairly large heart attack. Her son, Jose and daughter, Gladys, were by her bedside, and both were amazing. Soon, a grandson, Max, also arrived. Of the entire family, Max was the most grief-stricken.

I approached the family unrushed, and in a fashion entirely atypical of how I encounter patients with heart attack.

As I drove to the hospital, I had reflected carefully on this difficult situation. Would I do angioplasty if this had been my grandmother, I had been thinking.

What transpired thereafter is one of the many reasons I decided to write this book. I have thought long and hard about this case – to this date, I am not sure what the correct decision was and what it should be. Beyond the art and science of Medicine, the discipline may truly be an application of Philosophy. There is much that I learned through this overpowering experience. I continue to discuss this particular case with humility with so many other families in order to help them. This prudence will become transparent to you.

Irma's children, Jose and Gladys, had requested to speak with me. I too felt it was the most appropriate thing to do before making a rushed decision.

Astoundingly, their first question was remarkably lucid considering their circumstances, "Doctor, is she not too old to do this procedure?"

I was not certain of my answer, and I replied exactly so.

However, I hastened to patiently explain the likely scenario that would result from this heart attack. I explained to the family that there was a real possibility that left untreated; this heart attack could result in the demise of their mother.

I also informed them that I had indeed performed angioplasty on several patients in their 90s, and that most had done well. I told them that although the procedure would be difficult on account of Irma's frailty, it was not impossible.

Jose and Gladys listened patiently, but they could not decide. There were no easy answers. Max had also walked in, and his concerns were almost the same.

Gladys further inquired, "Doctor, we do have to make this decision fast, do we not?" I nodded in agreement but stated that this situation was different, and that they should discuss calmly and that I would wait for them to decide.

As I slowly got up to leave the room, Gladys asked again, this time even more directly, "Doctor, would you do this procedure if this was your mother?"

Deep in my heart, I knew this question was coming. To this day, I grope for the right answer. There probably is none, but what this remarkable family decided was as good   as any answer to this difficult question.

I witnessed myself this wonderful interaction. The emergency room was packed, but Irma was in a quiet cubicle. I sat a few feet away at the nursing desk, from where I witnessed these events unfold. The family went back to Irma after we spoke, and they explained to her about the heart attack. Both Gladys and Jose were in tears. Max was inconsolable. He simply could not bring words out of his mouth and kept hugging his grandmother. I was mesmerized by the calm disposition of this family.

Irma was speaking now. Clearly, she was halting and struggling. The scene was overwhelming – the ailing Irma was softly speaking, and Jose was gently stroking Irma's hair. Gladys rubbed her mother's hand, and Max bent over, sobbing.

A little while later, all three came out to speak to me. They were remarkably composed. Gladys, who had been the chosen spokeswoman, informed me that the family did not want the angioplasty procedure, and that they would accept whatever the outcome was from the heat attack.

After Gladys completed this statement, she looked at me questioningly. I put my hand gently on her shoulder and affirmed, "I think this is the right decision."

At 8:30 the next morning, Irma passed away.

The family never left her bedside, both in the emergency room and in her patient room. I learned later that the decision not to do angioplasty had been made by Irma. She had told the family that she was ready to go. She had lightheartedly told them that she had lived a long and good life and that she never expected to live 20 years longer than her husband.

Can you see yourself in any of these three situations? Do you believe that you may be confronted with any of these situations?

Before we dig deeper, let me quickly point out a very unusual commonality in these three patients. The presentations of these three elderly patients were atypical for an elderly patient who is having a heart attack. Several elderly patients, as we know, will not have any symptoms at all. The profound, crushing chest pain will be absent as will other classic manifestations. Commonly, the elderly may simply not feel well. They are often found to be lethargic or they offer vague complaints. Often, it requires great clinical acumen to recognize a heart attack in the elderly.

Medical ethics hold the immutable principle of respecting the patient's autonomy. However, when a patient's decision is not readily available, the family will confront a most challenging set of circumstances. There is extreme urgency in making critical, life- and-death decisions as it pertains to a heart attack. Sometimes, these decisions have life- long, emotional and psychological consequences. There is extreme stress that accompanies the shattering news of a loved one having a heart attack. It is understandable that this overwhelming event will cloud decision-making. As it is, verdicts regarding health and hospitalizations are difficult and complicated. Most patients struggle to make life- and-death decisions about their health, as they are emotionally vulnerable from the effects of pain and suffering. They will often lean on their spouse and family to help them in this decision.

Think back for a moment to when your loved one had to make a decision about undergoing a certain surgical procedure. Now, magnify this a hundred times and think how hard this can be if your loved one is having a heart attack, and you are called upon to make an instantaneous decision.

The cardiologist, as can be seen in these three cases, is also in a helpless position. Often, he or she will be asked for advice on these matters. By itself, this can be a challenging situation; it is made much worse by our prevailing medico-legal circumstances.

The situation of rushed decision-making in heart attacks deserves careful contemplation. Let us use the three cases to home in on the peculiar challenges of this decision-making.

In the case of Joyce, as there was no family available, Dr. Gupta and I had cosigned a "medical necessary" certificate. I performed the angioplasty, and the patient had a good outcome. The family was grateful. But what if poor Joyce had perforation of her artery while I was performing her angioplasty, or she needed emergency heart surgery? Worse, what if she died? How would the situation unfold with her family? Obviously, Elizabeth and Michael would be extremely upset.

Therefore, the urgent decision-making presents challenges to both the family and the physician. Death of a loved one is a catastrophic event. It is more severe when it occurs without notice. In these situations, the family is confronted with unbearable sorrow. This can translate into anger and guilt. Both these are acknowledged emotions in response to the death of a loved one. There is enormous anger and frustration at the system and with the providers. There may be immense remorse in not being involved in the decision- making and f or not being available when these tragic events were unfolding. The last is permanent. It is devastating. Blame is often assigned; retributions may be sought.

For a physician trying to provide life-saving care, this can be an awful situation. During my STEMI career, I have been inadvertently dragged into making critical and urgent decisions for elderly patients when their loved ones were not immediately available. This happened with Joyce. Imagine performing a complex and difficult procedure in circumstances without consent of the patient and knowledge of the family. Often, these are decisions made late in the night - with exhausted staff and with limited resources, not to mention, my own fatigue. Several of these circumstances concurred with Joyce. Fortunately, her outcome was excellent, but this should not take away from the adverse possibilities that may have unfolded. Often, physicians confront such challenges, and we are taught as a part of our medical ethics training how to deal with them. There are existent pathways of medical ethics and hospital committees that can help in such difficult situations. However, none may be available, late in the night, when confronted with similar situations in treating an elderly patient who is having a heart attack.

The situation with David and Norma was exceedingly complicated. David was incapacitated with the heart attack, and Norma was simply dazed and confused. The family was dysfunctional and a series of difficult decisions were made. Fortunately, in this case, they were made in consultation with numerous physicians and with some luxury of time. Both children abandoned the care of their parents when they needed it the most. Of course, this is extremely unfortunate, but it is not rare. I have confronted family members who openly and vociferously argue whether angioplasty should be performed for their elderly loved one. Some would strongly want angioplasty; others would forcefully disagree. Consensus may be difficult, and the urgency of the situation compounds this scenario.

Of course, a compassionate physician will greatly facilitate such choices, but even these earnest efforts can be thwarted by a multitude of very complex interactions and barriers that may be insurmountable in emergencies.

The last case history of Irma and her family is very profound.

As profound as the tragedy is, heart attacks may have a purpose in causing death of the very elderly.

However, its acceptance requires immense maturity.

This remarkable family understood the true meaning of life and purpose of death. How many physicians wish they could confront such great families in their difficult decision-making.

As I have previously admitted, I still struggle with what my decision would have been if Irma were my grandmother?

As a cardiologist, I know I could abort her heart attack, but as a grandson, I cannot see her suffer.

Heart attack is a fairly quick and relatively pain-free end of life. This awful statement is terrible but it is a truthful and painful admission that I make.

Irma was 97; she had lived a good life. The family made a collaborative decision, and the heart attack resulted in uncomplicated demise. Of course, this raises so many difficult and unanswerable questions. As I write this book, I tend to lean towards this decision for my loved one. But it would be burdening.

A clearer answer is that if this were to be me as the patient - passing away from a heart attack at 97? I would take it any day.

How to define "elderly" remains difficult. We understand that the chronological age is an oversimplification. The patient's functional level is a more appropriate response. Patients are healthy and living independently into the nineties. At this "elderly" age, they are autonomous, still driving, and living remarkable, vigorous lives.

Who are we to call anybody "elderly?"

There is truly no age cutoff.

However, this situation becomes complicated when elderly patients lose their spouse. We have all seen our loved ones age dramatically after losing a spouse.

For the purpose of decision-making regarding heart attacks, I leave it to the reader to come up with their own definition – is their loved one elderly?

Let's now provide you with some guiding principles in managing the care and decision-making of your elderly parent or grandparent.

1. Anticipate these situations. Specifically, concentrate on individual elderly loved ones. Do they live alone? Whom should they contact? How can you be reached? Who else can be included in the decision-making? Obtain a clear living will if possible.

2. For each elderly loved one, collaboratively assign a decision plan if they were to have a heart attack. Consult with their doctor ahead of time about these decisions.

3. Establish clearly if their life will have meaningful existence after the angioplasty.

CHAPTER 9. CAN I PREVENT A HEART ATTACK?

Giving up smoking is the easiest thing in the world. I know
because I've done it thousands of times.
Mark Twain

Here comes the real value for the time spent in reading this book.

After all, what is the use of gaining so much wisdom about heart attacks and not being able to prevent one? I am not going to make any claims that I am an absolute expert in this area, but there is none. This is an evolving field in which considerable research is occurring. There are no magic pills. At least, I have possibly the world's largest experience in treating patients who are having a heart attack. I have also had the humility to observe the lifestyles of hundreds of these patients who were having a heart attack. Through these careful observations, a very clear pattern of self-neglect emerges. There is so much that can be learned from these painstaking observations and from my decades of work treating thousands of patients with heart attacks.

I must quickly confess that there will be some personal bias in my recommendations; however, I will also balance these sanctions with prudent scientific facts and guidelines.

Almost every patient who has a heart attack should go into a cardiac rehab program. Strictly defined, a cardiac rehab is a medically supervised program that helps improve the health and wellbeing of people who have heart problems, including a heart attack. Rehab programs include exercise-training, education about heart healthy living, and counseling to reduce stress, and help you to return to an active life. Although the number of patients who are seeking cardiac rehab is increasing, less than 1/3 of patients who sustained a heart attack enroll in a cardiac rehab program. Besides strongly advocating enrollment in a cardiac rehab program, I want to instill fundamental education about the individual risk factors.

Coronary artery disease and heart attacks are primarily end results of uncontrolled risk factors. This is not news, but every risk factor does not necessarily have equal weight, in the context of our present-day lifestyle. Let us go into the specifics.

To recap, the traditional risk factors for heart attacks are diabetes, high blood pressure, smoking, and high lipids. These are the four big traditional risk factors. In addition to these, the male sex, stress, family history, and perhaps pollution, are also contributing factors. These add up to eight total risk factors. Several researchers will point to additional risk factors. Let us address each individually and understand its relative importance.

As far as avoiding risk factors go, the one that is absolutely mandatory is a complete cessation of smoking. Period. There is no half-truth here. Neither are there shortcuts. On this critical matter, there simply can be no argument. If you have had a heart attack, you absolutely must give up smoking. If you want to prevent a heart attack, my recommendation is equally emphatic. With smoking, it is not a matter of how you will have coronary artery disease or a heart attack, it is only when. The noxious influence of nicotine on the heart, whether the source is cigarettes, cigar, electronic cigarettes, or chewing tobacco, produces the same end result. There is undisputed and overwhelming scientific evidence that demonstrates how destructive the effect of nicotine is on the coronary artery, coronary plaque, the endothelial lining, and the coronary stent. In short, every aspect that causes heart attacks is promoted by nicotine. These severe injuries to the heart are progressive and accelerating.

Smoking after treatment of a heart attack promotes rapid re-accumulation of thrombus on the steel mesh of the coronary stent. It virtually takes away the benefits that come from aspirin and other newer antiplatelet agents. By continuing to smoke, there is both a quashing of the benefits of life-saving drugs and a further progression of disease. There should be absolutely no doubt in the mind of a patient who has had a heart attack that smoking needs to be *immediately* stopped.

A heart attack is a life-changing event. People remember this for their entire life, and some recollect this as "when I almost died." This frightening experience presents a fantastic opportunity to kill a habit that has persisted. In the years that I have performed the amazing procedure of angioplasty to treat heart attacks, I have encountered hundreds of patients who were willing to give up anything in return for surviving from the heart attack. Medical students are taught that heart attack patients have severe chest pain, difficulty in breathing, sweating, and fainting. All correct. In addition, what most patients feel is an absolute fear of death.

Suddenly, these patients are not invincible. Their bravado about their smoking habit is now shattered. Suddenly, they are willing to give up something that previously felt impossible. And suddenly, the physician is presented with the fantastic opportunity to break a deadly addiction.

The physician must immediately grab this opportunity to help the patient. Of course, I will also address patients who have not had a heart attack. First, let us try to prevent a second heart attack for a smoker who continues to unwisely smoke after surviving a heart attack.

One of the misfortunes of medical advances is that treatment for numerous medical conditions has become too easy. Patients with a heart attack used to stay in the hospital for two weeks, after which they had months of gradual rehabilitation. My patients with a heart attack are now going home on the second day after their angioplasty. It is simply too easy. They have been spared the prolonged agony of a long and expensive hospitalization and extremely slow recovery from a heart attack. The oversimplification can lead to complacency. Yet, overwhelmingly, patients will respond to interventions about smoking cessation at this critical juncture when they have just experienced a heart attack. This experience is simply too frightening; even the most stoic patient is rattled. What is critically needed is for the family and physician to firmly intervene at this precious juncture. Several patients will go complete cold turkey at this instance. This is fantastic. I only wish this horrendous feel permeated in the mind of every patient whom I treat for a heart attack. I wish there becomes a legal path for a patient signing a pledge to give up smoking if he survives a heart attack. These impossibilities notwithstanding, an absolute mandate must be placed by the physician on this patient to immediately quit smoking. In this regard, the few early weeks after heart attack treatment are invaluable to break the smoking habit. Some patients will quit completely, but almost all of them will consider quitting. This superb progress can be greatly supported by instituting nicotine substitutes such as chewing gum. Call me old-fashioned, or too rigid but I firmly believe that a heart attack survivor will go cold turkey with forceful intervention. The patient has witnessed a completely shattering assault to the notion that he or she could get away with smoking.

The heart attack is a game changer for smokers. The worst smoking addicts have, perhaps for the first time, faced a near-death experience brought upon by their smoking addiction. They are now willing to quit this habit and they may permanently rid themselves of it. Although smokers will have other contributing factors, there is no question that smoking is the most immediately modifiable factor.

In my immediate interaction with smokers who have had heart attacks, I am relentless in my sanctions about smoking. There are no halfway solutions in this moment of life and death. I am completely convinced about the correctness of this firm stance. Therefore, my advice to the patient is unambiguous. They must stop smoking immediately. I completely squash any bargaining that the patient offers, "I will give it up soon," or "I just need some time to take care of it," or worse, "can I do it slowly?" No, you cannot do it slowly. You cannot give up smoking over the next few months. This is completely unacceptable, and it is the absolutely correct recommendation for the patient. This immutable mandate must be expressed by the patients' loved ones too. Any vacillation about this by family members only weakens the patient's resolve at the time when the patient   is willing to change. I have also encountered a disturbing and bizarre phenomenon. The smoker who survived a heart attack is made complacent by another smoking loved one. In many ways, what I am writing about constitutes family therapy. However, despite this being the scenario, I want to maintain focus on the smoker who has just survived the heart attack. Here is a small, final anecdote. Fernando Vasquez, 47, lifelong smoker survived a massive heart attack. His wife, Linda threatened to file for divorce if Fernando kept smoking. Many would find this as extreme, which it probably is. Yet, the intent is correct, and the wife's conduct is motivated by sincerity and love.

The role of immediate family members, including the spouse and the children, is paramount in the early period after the heart attack. The family must collectively deliver this firm and sustained message. No complacency on this matter is acceptable.

Almost always, after finishing the heart attack angioplasty, as I deliver the good news to the loved ones of the patient surviving the heart attack, I quickly seize this opportunity to emphasize this critical intervention. Often, the family is not even available before the procedure as EMS brought the patient alone. Doctors in the emergency room have often obtained the consent. Of course, I am always available and willing to answer any questions that the patient or the family has prior to the procedure. Most patients, however, are simply asking for pain relief pleading for intervention. It is mainly after the procedure that I begin to address risk factors.

Having done this for so many years, I recognize that the opportunity to modify risk factors is not in the immediate aftermath of angioplasty. However, it is the most opportune moment to specifically address smoking.

I have never insulted a suffering patient, who is on the catheterization table, by reprimanding him or her about smoking. I have, at times, addressed this immediately after the procedure, even with the patient, before going out to speak to the family members. I emphasize again that this is a unique moment to helping the patient to stop smoking.

My practiced art of recommending risk factor modification therefore falls into two stages. In the first stage, immediately after the angioplasty, and when the horror of the heart attack is fresh, I meticulously address smoking. Other risk factors can be discussed later. Tonight, in the immediate aftermath of surviving a heart attack, is the moment to seize. Of course, I am smart enough to not let this be further stressful for a vulnerable patient. But, this is not a bargaining moment. By selflessly and skillfully saving a patient's life, I have earned a capital of trust and confidence that I want to trade for smoking cessation altogether by the patient. I have only the patient's best interest in my heart. The patient has had a second chance, and I want to prevent another catastrophic event.

For a patient who has not had a heart attack, this chapter should be a forewarning of your fate. You risk having a heart attack and everything in your life by continuing to smoke. Anything you can do to quit smoking is appropriate. Get every counseling that you need, every substitute you can find, but quit. Nowhere am I suggesting that this will be easy. Often this is an addiction that spanned decades. The good news is that once you stop smoking, the benefits begin fairly quickly. By one year after quitting, you have almost eliminated this terrible risk factor.

There is one more topic of intense controversy that I wish to discuss. It is regarding insurance coverage for smokers, in particular, those who have survived a heart attack. In certain countries, such as the United Kingdom, the National Health Services could conceivably deny medical coverage for smokers. Of course, this is hypothetical, but it is conceivable. Smokers increase the adversity of the risk pool of insured members. Perhaps, we need to consider a stricter deterrent for smokers, in particular, those who have survived a heart attack.

I will address the next three big factors together. These include diabetes, high blood pressure, and high lipids. In some ways, the remedy for these risk factors is also applicable to stress. There is no substitute to good medical therapy and counseling from the primary care physician for these risk factors. Diabetes, as we have discussed in earlier chapters, is of two types, one that requires insulin and one that does not.

The insulin-dependent variety is more virulent and will often require specialized care provided by an endocrinologist. The type of insulin and its precise dose and timing are critical. The use of novel modes of administration, including the insulin pump, also requires careful evaluation. Surveillance of blood glucose levels is paramount. These are all highly specialized functions that need fairly regular expert handling by a specialist. Of critical importance is for the diabetic to understand that the ill effects of diabetes result from sustained and elevated blood glucose levels. A well-regulated blood glucose level instituted through a rigidly monitored insulin strategy is the most scientific way to minimize and delay the harmful effects of diabetes on the heart. The situation for the non-insulin dependent diabetes patient is mostly along the same lines. Fortunately, these patients are spared the absolute requirement of regular insulin therapy. However, this group of diabetics require careful monitoring and it would be a miscalculation to let complacency creep into their management. It is important to maintain adequate and lowered blood glucose level for this group too. Fortunately, with oral agents and through dietary controls, this less severe form of diabetes can be controlled.

There is an important caveat, which is that the non-insulin group can degenerate into requiring insulin at a later stage, hence the increased need of surveillance for the non- insulin group.

Both groups of diabetes patients, unfortunately, require lifelong surveillance of their conditions.

High blood pressure puts stress on the major arteries of the body, including the aorta, the biggest blood vessel in our body. It also imposes stress on the pumping chambers of the heart, the left ventricle. In addition to heart attacks, persistently elevated blood pressure increases the risk of stroke. Failure of the heart muscle is another deadly, long-term complication. Almost every decade has witnessed the lowering of blood pressure targets, as instituted by the American Heart Association. Most patients will require drug therapy, often with multiple agents. There is enormous variability in these drugs, with several being more advantageous depending on age, sex, and race. Most internists can select the most appropriate blood pressure regimen. As with blood glucose levels, long-term control of the blood pressure is the goal.

In an earlier part of the book, I discussed the good and bad cholesterol as well as triglycerides. Major improvement of the lipid equilibrium can be achieved with statins. These powerful agents are extremely effective in lowering the bad cholesterol, or LDL, as well as in raising the good cholesterol, or HDL. They also have an amazing effect of preventing the inflammatory component that leads to "plaque rupture," the initial physiological change that leads to a heart attack. Most of the newer statin drugs are extremely predictable in their response – this adds to their remarkable effectiveness in lowering the levels. It is possible to fairly accurately predict how much reduction in LDL can be obtained through these agents as well as the approximate HDL increases. The use of statins has become a mainstay in the treatment of heart disease. Approximately 25 million Americans are now taking a statin drug (familiar brand names include Lipitor, Crestor, Vytorin, and Zocor). By a recent calculation, another 13 million Americans could benefit from these drugs. However, these drugs are not without their associated problems. Up to 20% of these patients are deemed statin intolerant. These patients experience significant side effects that often require dose reduction, switching to another agent, or stopping the drug altogether. Their symptoms include muscle aches in the arms, shoulders, thighs, or hips, generalized weakness, gastrointestinal symptoms, and liver problems.

Let us briefly also review the prevalence of the individual risk factors. This would explain my obsession about risk factor modification. Approximately 100 million Americans have elevated lipids! 70 million Americans have high blood pressure! There are 25 million diabetics and 40 million smokers! Of course, several of these risk factors are overlapping. Irrespective, we face an epidemic of coronary artery disease risk factors.

Let me now provide the common denominator to reduce blood

pressure, lipids, stress, and to manage diabetes. It is by exercise. Exercise, in my assessment, is the single best antidote to coronary artery disease. It even has indirect benefits for smokers. For its role in reducing multiple risk factors simultaneously, the benefits of exercise are paramount. I will therefore address it comprehensively.

Let me first announce that I live the life that I preach. There are virtually no days in my personal life when I do not exercise. I have maintained almost the same blood pressure, blood cholesterol, and weight in the last 25 years. It will remain my sincere endeavor to maintain these levels over the next few decades too. I have been blessed not to have diabetes, high blood pressure, or familial lipid disorders, and I have never smoked. This is a minor and insignificant detail by most standards, but it is important for me, as I have always maintained that I must set a personal example for my patients.

It is important to understand the coronary physiology and some important attributes of the arteries that supply the heart. This knowledge is not required for the ordinary patient, but I offer it to the scientist in you. We have always focused on the three major coronary arteries. These three arteries lie on the surface of the heart, and we call them epicardial coronary arteries. In addition to these three major coronary arteries, there are hundreds of small branches and smaller vessels known as the capillaries. In essence, the heart is a vascular bed supplied by countless numbers of these micro vessels that permeate the heart muscle. An extremely well-conditioned heart is supplied with these numerous blood vessels. In a well-perfused heart, the presence of numerous small vessels supplements the flow from the major epicardial vessels. In a patient with heart attack, these additional vessels are recruited to supply blood to the dying or "necrosing" muscle cells. These recruited vessels, or coronary collaterals, often contribute to sustaining life during a heart attack. The role of exercise is to develop this intracardiac network of blood vessels. Just like exercise promotes muscle tone, these vessels become more abundant and perfused with exercise. In a patient who exercises regularly, these vessels are protective during a heart attack. For a patient after a heart attack, it is the recruitment of these additional vessels that contributes to cardiac well-being.

Exercise is of two major forms, isotonic and isometric. Isometric exercise is a type of strengthening exercise in which the joint angle and muscle length do not change during contraction. Isotonic exercises, also known as dynamic constant external resistance (DCER), include exercises where muscle tendons pull against bones to cause joint movement. Weight training, rowing, and running fall into the isotonic category. In fitness, isotonic exercise most commonly refers to exercises that isolate a particular muscle group to increase strength or improve performance.

Since most human activity and athletic performance involve movement, isotonic exercise is the basis of most training protocols, as it emphasizes muscle contraction for motion more than resistance. Examples include walking, running, and sports such as golf, tennis, swimming, soccer, baseball, and most calisthenics. Isotonic exercises tend to raise the heart rate more than the blood pressure. These exercises lead to slimmer and longer muscle. Swimmers and runners look different than weight lifters. Isotonic exercise is often called "cardio" as it is good for cardiac conditioning.

I hope I have convinced my audience about the benefits of exercise. There are a few practical tips. The most frequent questions about exercise that patients ask me after their heart attack are - which exercises should they do, how often, and how much?

Before answering these questions, there is a more important issue: when should exercise commence after a heart attack? Ordinarily, in most circumstances, two weeks after a heart attack is when patients can return to work and enroll themselves into a cardiac rehab program. By the same token, beginning exercise gradually two weeks after a heart attack is often recommended. We are mainly dealing with isotonic exercises after a heart attack. These will contribute to developing a more perfused heart and offer enormous benefits for the control of diabetes, blood pressure, lipids, stress, and smoking. This sentence is deliberately repeated to emphasize the multiple benefits of exercise for simultaneous reduction of multiple risk factors.

As a practical point, it should be an exercise that is sustainable and enjoyable. Intense regimens will often become boring and not durable. A very common trend is for the enthusiastic heart attack survivor to head into an exhausting workout routine that cannot be sustained.

The essence of risk factor control after a heart attack is lifestyle modification. I believe that adoption of a middle path (as depicted in Buddhism) may offer a balanced approach. It is an altered and corrupted lifestyle with occurrence of numerous risk factors that contributes to a heart attack. This book is not an effort to discuss philosophy or to have religious undertones. I will clearly stay off these elements except where I feel they directly contribute to a patient's emotional and psychological wellbeing. Clearly, some of these cultural, religious, and spiritual beliefs will manifest in patients' lives, often, in more ways than we directly admit. It is often decades of unhealthy living that contributes to unmitigated risk factors that cause a heart attack. Many patients are obese and have sedentary lifestyles; many are couch potatoes, and many are consumers of diets rich in saturated fats. This pattern has been ongoing for decades, and it requires a systematic evaluation. Counseling and cardiac rehab greatly contribute to this assessment and management. Although cardiac rehab programs are recommended for most patients after a heart attack, genuine lifestyle modification is an individual responsibility beyond admittance into a program. It begins with a sensible and an honest acceptance of these lifestyle-draining factors. Self-denial hugely distorts a sensible, astute, and honest assessment. It often requires very patient appraisal for patients to accurately identify where their lifestyle became extreme.

Therefore, the question which exercise, how and when - is answered by the sole purpose of exercise as being a great modifier of one's lifestyle.

One should choose a form of exercise that can be sustained, and which is a prudent lifestyle adjustment. It is ridiculous to expect a 68-year-old patient, who was previously sedentary, to become a runner after his heart attack. This has to be a gradual lifestyle change that the patient understands and can sustain. Unless this behavioral change is maintained, its benefits will be temporary. That would defeat the purpose of risk factor modification. Therefore, in counseling lifestyle modification, I carefully assess a patient's lifestyle. In doing so, it becomes readily apparent which form of exercise and its duration should be offered to a particular patient.

Many patients will gain sustainable benefit from regular walking. Of these, the most that are helped are elderly patients who cannot be expected to have intense athletic pursuits. However, regular daily walking, often with the spouse, has numerous benefits. Beyond its cardiovascular enhancement, such relaxed, but disciplined routine, is also stress relieving. It has the added benefit of enhancing good health for the entire family. In many ways, the family participates in the patient's exercise regimen. Of course, running, biking, and swimming are fantastic options. Of all these, none compares to the benefits of swimming, as the exercise is the most physiological. For patients who can swim and have a good facility where they can swim regularly, this remains my top recommendation.

The duration of exercise can be calculated easily, and it places emphasis on achieving a target heart rate during exercise. As stated before, isotonic exercises benefit the heart more than isometric exercise. With improved cardiac performance, the heart rate lowers in response to exercise. Well-conditioned athletes have heart rates in the 40-50s. One of the easy and practical ways to document your cardiac performance is by monitoring your heart rate. With gradual and regular exercise, you are able to lower your heart rate, both at rest and during exercise. Since the heart rate is controlled by various other bodily elements, in ways, this is an oversimplification, but it is an inexpensive way to gauge your progress. Several easy to use heart rate monitors are available and they may be used beneficially.

The formula for calculating the duration of exercise is as follows: the heart rate that you should achieve with exercise is calculated as 85% of (220 − age). This target heart rate should then be maintained for 20 minutes with exercise. This regimen should be followed at least three times a week.

Let us make this simple. Let us assume your age is 60. Then, according to this simple formula, 220-60 = 160. 85% of this is 136 beats per minute. So, purely by physiological definition, cardio fitness for this patient is defined as maintaining a heart rate of 136 beats per minutes for at least 20 minutes, irrespective of the mode of exercise. This can be achieved by any of the following isotonic exercises such as walking jogging running, cycling, swimming, and sports.

Beyond these scientific calculations, a pragmatic approach is to advocate the activity that can be sustained. As I suggested before, this activity should be incorporated as a lifestyle modification. If it is seen as a mere temporary resolve as a result of the heart attack, it will not fulfill its larger aim.

Almost the same discipline is needed to make dietary changes. Many years ago, I used to be a very strong advocate for making intense and rigorous dietary restrictions. Of course, I still maintain that common dietary excursions such as red meat, whole milk, cheese, egg yolk, and fried foods, must be avoided. Yet, I have backed off from extreme rigidity in my views based upon the profound benefits of statins that are being used by almost all patients following their heart attacks. The use of statins is a strict guideline recommendation by the American Heart Association for all patients who have had heart attacks. The statins make a much greater dent in the levels of lipids than by the individual reduction of common food items. However, several patients will not be able to tolerate these drugs, and dietary modifications are critical. Counseling, as and when needed, is required.

When I review the two, exercise and diet, I firmly conclude that the overwhelming benefits of exercise rule supreme. I am not advocating any dietary digressions. Instead, they have to be complementary. However, exercise should be the fundamental basis of risk factor modification.

The last item that needs deep thought is meditation – pun intended. Before eschewing the benefits of meditation, let us understand the science of stress.

Exercise is a powerful anti-stress activity. In fact, one of the biggest benefits of exercise is its reduction of stress levels. Patients and individuals routinely express a feeling of wellbeing with exercise. This is an indisputable scientific fact. The level of blood hormones, or catecholamine, rises during stress. These levels are reduced with exercise and relaxing techniques. The catecholamine greatly contributes to an unhealthy heart and body. They result in elevated blood pressure, heart rate, and their levels have been recognized   to adversely affect blood sugar and lipids levels.

Let us now examine the relaxing techniques that can reduce stress and catecholamine levels. These techniques have become a vogue, and yoga is now a part of the American life. Irrespective, meditation has profound scientific merits. Over the last decade, its beneficial effects have been systematically studied. Most relate to the specific decrease of catecholamine levels.

On a deeper level, yoga is a form of meditation. Various meditation techniques such as transcendental meditation (TM) have been individually studied and they demonstrate numerous benefits for the heart. I strongly advocate these techniques for patients after they have sustained a heart attack. Even for normal and healthy individuals, they can only benefit. A practical difficulty is choosing a good teacher who can teach these relaxing techniques.

I strongly urge you to find that teacher.

CHAPTER 10. IN CONCLUSION

Learn from yesterday, live for today, hope for tomorrow. The important thing is not to stop questioning.
Albert Einstein

We are blessed in the United States that heart attacks, which previously killed so many of us, are less deadly now. Most of us will receive quick, early treatment and survive the heart attack. This book has attempted to provide a checklist of early recognition, management, and prevention of heart attacks.

Several new developments are going to further improve the STEMI process and procedure. We can expect better stents and drugs. A further simplification of the convoluted STEMI process will also occur. Beyond educating my audience, it has been a deliberate exercise that I conducted through this book to raise social awareness about existent flaws in the system. In particular, the public reporting of STEMI statistics and the individual ranking of hospitals and physicians that treat these patients must be objective and not simply billboard pronouncements of "best heart attack center."

An educated patient will most likely have a better outcome, and I hope I have provided you this knowledge.

It may be prudent for us to step back and realize how fortunate we are in this country. The rest of the world is struggling trying to create systems that can treat heart attacks and millions in developing countries will die from a heart attack before this book is even published! This is truly unfortunate. We are simply too slow in globally adopting the seismic scientific advancements for treating heart attacks with angioplasty. In 2019, patients should not die from a heart attack anywhere. It should bother the conscience of every cardiologist that a young man or woman dies anywhere in the world from a heart attack. Primary angioplasty that treats patients with heart attacks is one of the biggest scientific advancements of this century. Its predictability in dramatically opening the occluded coronary artery is dazzling. This technique must be made available to patients worldwide, immediately.

This is the task of my Lumen Foundation that is uncompromisingly dedicated to saving lives from AMI. Already, various techniques and strategies that were developed at this organization are essential components of heart attack management in numerous poor countries. I sincerely hope that this work can gain further steam, and that numerous other organizations coalesce to make this a global endeavor.

As exemplified with the Peace Corps, the United States has always taken a lead in advancing global progress. This is most demonstrable in medical sciences. American inventions have led the way in improving healthcare around the world. Along the way, American technology has been a fantastic partner in the advancement of medical sciences. American physicians have contributed their time to help patients worldwide for decades.

It is now time for us to advance angioplasty for the benefit of mankind. We can all help. Unexpectedly, my most passionate plea goes to social media. We can powerfully, speedily and cost-effectively spread the message of awareness about heart attack management and prevention through social media. Imagine the global power of this book if parts of it resonate on Facebook and Twitter. The powerful message and sincere recommendations could reach millions instantaneously. At the foundation of heart attack management is public awareness. Social media can make primary angioplasty a global movement. Foremost, it will do so by increasing patient awareness.

Upon reading this book, you would have recognized my passion for Primary PCI. I believe I am the only cardiologist in the world that has performed STEMI Interventions as a dedicated occupation for over 15 years. In the early years of this historic pursuit, I first spent several years mastering the STEMI procedure and in creating innovative techniques to improve outcomes. Then, I systematically improved the STEMI procedure. In the process, I convinced myself, and physicians that followed my work, about the need to improve both the STEMI procedure and the process. It was obvious that improving the STEMI process was the harder challenge. The last few years have been audacious exercises in taking this message global. The Lumen Global meeting, the annual scientific deliberations of the philanthropic Lumen Foundation, is held in a different world capital each year. Over the years, this meeting has dented barriers to urgent heart attack management.

I firmly believe that by itself the powerful engine of angioplasty is unstoppable. Lumen Foundation is a mere catalyst that is thrusting forward this powerful dispatch. Catheterization laboratories are emerging in the poorest parts of the world, and their most common procedure is to treat patients with heart attack. Thousands of young cardiologists recognize this groundbreaking technique, towards which they are passionately committed. Lumen Global is training these physicians, several hundred each year. It is also creating important local stakeholders. In 2013, in India, the Lumen Global "meeting" became a "movement." Social media can exponentially grow this movement.

No longer should bureaucrats and politicians be able to deny this fantastic procedure to millions of patients who have heart attacks. Too many parts of the world are lacking in the infrastructure and resources for developing cath labs. They struggle with less effective alternatives of treating heart attacks, such as thrombolytic therapy. I have never denied the tremendous contributions and accessibility of thrombolytic therapy, but if I am having a heart attack, I prefer angioplasty with a short Door-to-Balloon time.

I conclude this book with a mention of two important subjects. I emphatically believe that telemedicine can facilitate access to heart attack care in poor countries. Hopefully, its technological advancement and its supplementation with additional funding will catapult this methodology. The Lumen Foundation has populated vast regions in Brazil and Colombia with telemedicine. Remote cardiologists accurately diagnose heart attacks and tele consult the patient's management. With this methodology, 42% of Colombia's 48 million patients now have access to telemedicine as a part of the Latin America Telemedicine Infarct Network (LATIN) program. A total of 104 telemedicine centers are now active in Colombia and Brazil. This program is now being advanced to Mexico. Variants of this program have recently provided a telemedicine-STEMI umbrella to the 65 million inhabitants of India's largest state, Rajasthan. To me, telemedicine appears the technology to provide cost-effective heart attack management to vast populations, in particular, in poor African, Latin American, and Asian countries.

The next enterprise pertains to women and it intends to dent the higher death rates that women experience when they have heart attacks, including in the United States. It is ironic that a nation that prepares to elect its first female President has not normalized gender differences in heart attack. The Lumen Foundation also recognizes that there are centuries-old personal, social, cultural, financial, and religious barriers that cannot be overcome in the rushed urgency of a heart attack. We must overcome these barriers. An effective tool available for us to eliminate these disparities, in 2019, is social media.

Good luck with your heart attack! You will survive.

ACKNOWLEDGMENT

Over the last 15 years, the following research fellows have greatly contributed to my work. I thank them.

H. *Aboushi* MD	A. *Hidalgo* MD	L. *Pisana* MD
M. *Acosta* MD	V. *Jorapur* MD	J. *Pratt*
J. *Aguilar* MD	V. *Herrera* MD	S. *Quintero* MD
C. *Alfonso* MD	A. *Ishmael* MD	O. *Reynbakh* MD
R. *Bakhtiani*	R. *Jacobucci* MD	D. *Rodríguez* MD
M. *Bhatt* MD	J. *Kostala* MD	R. *Rowen* MD
R. *Briceño* MD	S. *Krisciunas* MD	R. *Safie* MD
M. *Castillo* MD	M. *Lifleur*	F. *Shamshad* MD
C. *Cárdenas*	C. *Lopez* MD	S. *Sunkaraneni* MD
E. *Cecilio* MD	Y. *Ma*	M. *Torres* MD
M. *Ceschim*	J. *Mazzini* MD	K. *Treto* MD
S. *Cohen* MD	N. *Meza-Ruiz* MD	I. *Vallenilla* MD
Z. *Dahya* MD	P. *Moyer*	A. *Velásquez* MD
J. *Day*	M. *Marin* MD	D. *Vieira* MD
P. *Del Toro*	A. *Munguia* MD	T. *Waisman* MD
B. *Falcao* MD	M. *Narang* MD	S. *Yebara* MD
E. *Falcao* MD	F. *Nola*	P. *Yépez* MD
A. *Ferré* MD	E. *Oliveros* MD	N. *Yousef*
F. *Fernández*	M. *Ossa*	T. *Zhang* B.S.
A. *Frauenfelder* MD	C. *Peña*	D. *Zwakenberg* MD
A. *Flores* MD	F. *Pérez* MD	
C. *Funatsu* MD	G. *Pinto* MD	

Four of these individuals deserve additional credit, Dr. Rosanna Briceño, for creating the SINCERE database, Dr. Maria Monica Ossa for helping write LATIN protocols, Dr. Alexandra Ferré for assisting with GLOW, and Tracy Zhang, for overseeing the entire construction of this book.

...AND SURVIVING IT

GLOSSARY

AMI: Acute Myocardial Infarction. A heart attack.

Artery: a blood vessel that carries oxygenated blood to vital organs.

Atherosclerosis: the diffuse disease that is seen in various arteries that manifest with blockages. It results from presence of risk factors.

CAD: Coronary Artery Disease. Blockages in one of the three major arteries that supply the heart muscle.

Cardiac Catheterization: the diagnostic procedure performed to find blockages in the coronary arteries.

CATH Lab: dedicated place in a hospital, where specialized heart invasive procedures are performed, such as PCI.

D2B Time: Door to Balloon Time. The precise time, in minutes, that is counted from the time when a patient with a heart attack enters the emergency room, until the time when his blocked coronary artery is opened.

EKG: Electrocardiogram. Electrical recording of the heart that is used to diagnose various heart abnormalities.

EMS: Emergency Medical Services, responsible for ambulance care.

ER: Emergency Room.

Left Ventricle: the pumping chamber of the heart.

Lipids: types of fat that are deposited in blood vessels.

LMCA: Left Main Coronary Artery. The big trunk that supplies blood to the heart muscle. It has two branches, the Left Anterior Descendant (LAD) and the Left Circumflex (LCx).

Paramedics: skilled persons that care for a patient in an ambulance.

PCI: Percutaneous Coronary Intervention. The collection of various procedures used to treat blockages in coronary arteries. This list includes balloons, stents, cutting devices, laser and use of radiation.

RCA: Right Coronary Artery.

STEMI Intervention: the procedure to urgently open occluded coronary arteries during a heart attack.

STEMI: ST elevation myocardial infarction. The most severe form of heart attack that requires urgent treatment.

Stents: metallic scaphoid that is inserted into the coronary artery to treat blockages.

Stress Test: a treadmill test that monitors the function of the heart during exercise.

Telemedicine: management of a disease by experts that are remotely located.

Vein: a blood vessel that takes deoxygenated blood from the vital organs to the heart.

VF: Ventricular Fibrillation. The most critical heart rhythm irregularity that can be fatal if not treated urgently.

VT: Ventricular Tachycardia. A dangerous irregularity of the heart rhythm that can be seen during a heart attack.

Made in the USA
Columbia, SC
26 July 2019